ALSO BY MAX LERNER

It Is Later Than You Think
Ideas Are Weapons
Ideas for the Ice Age
The Mind and Faith of Justice Holmes
Public Journal
The Portable Veblen
Actions and Passions
America as a Civilization
The Unfinished Country
The Age of Overkill
Education and a Radical Humanism
Tocqueville and American Civilization
Values in Education
Ted and the Kennedy Legend

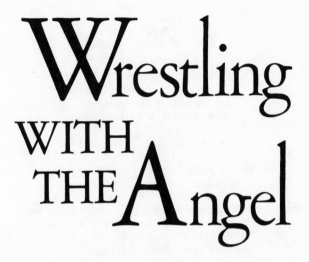

Wrestling WITH THE Angel

A Memoir of My Triumph over Illness

MAX LERNER

A TOUCHSTONE BOOK
Published by Simon & Schuster
New York   London   Toronto   Sydney   Tokyo   Singapore

TOUCHSTONE
Simon & Schuster Building
Rockefeller Center
1230 Avenue of the Americas
New York, New York 10020

First Touchstone Edition 1991
Published by arrangement with W. W. Norton & Company,
500 Fifth Avenue, New York, New York 10110
TOUCHSTONE and colophon are registered trademarks
of Simon & Schuster Inc.
Manufactured in the United States of America

1 3 5 7 9 10 8 6 4 2 Pbk.

Library of Congress Cataloging in Publication Data
Lerner, Max, date.
Wrestling with the angel: a memoir of my triumph over illness/
Max Lerner. — 1st Touchstone ed.
p. cm.
"A Touchstone book."
Previously published: New York: Norton, © 1990.
Includes bibliographical references (p.   ).
1. Lerner, Max, date.—Health. 2. Cancer—Patients—United
States—Biography. 3. Heart—Infarction—Patients—United
States—Biography. I. Title.
RC265.6.L47A3 1991
362.1′96994′0092—dc20
[B]   91-7943
CIP
ISBN 0-671-74095-4 Pbk.

For Jenny
—and for my children
Adam, Stephen, Michael, Joanna, Constance,
who are in the camp of life

And in memory of
my daughter Pamela Schofield
who died of cancer at 29

CONTENTS

Author's Note 11

1. Contingency Is King 19

2. The Locus of the Evil 27

3. The Torment of Choice 37

4. The Universe of the Ill 47

5. Don't Take My Night Away 59

6. "You Are Twice-Blessed: You Have Two Cancers" 77

7. "Don't Let Them Do an Abelard on You" 95

8. A Medical Miracle—and a Medical Museum 111

9. "Thank God, It's Only a Heart Attack!" 117

10. The Upward Spiral: The Doctor Within the Patient 137

11. Aging: The Last Voyage 145

12. Confronting Death, Asserting Life 167

Notes 196

Further Reading 205

AUTHOR'S NOTE

THESE PAGES are a narrative of a life-threatening illness. I have seen it through a patient's eye, not a doctor's, which is bound to make a difference. I shall be telling of two successive cancers, followed by a heart attack, all in the space of four or five years. For a time I felt like Job.

My first cancer came when I was seventy-eight, and after a year the prognosis was pretty dark. But I learned that command belongs to the patient, and made a fight of it, as I did of the two successor episodes. I was lucky in the doctors who worked with me, and in the cohesiveness of my large and supportive family.

Since I am by profession a writing man, not certain whether something has happened until I can put it into words, I kept a fitful account of my adventures in ailing and healing—and of my aging as well, although I tend to regard the ailing/aging complex as an unholy alliance.

Consequently I have ventured, at various points, to flesh out the bare bones of the narrative by inserting journal entries, some of them written in the full flood of feeling and of narcissism, with little concern for the niceties of language or the imperatives of modesty. Some others are more reflective, at times even meditative, as I try in my journals to give an account to myself of the complex role of the shaman in the doctor–patient relation, the intricacies and uncertainties of the mind–body connection, the miseries and splendors of the aging experience, the dialectical dances of life and death, and even some explorations of the presence of God in the one-sided conversations I started with Him.

For the metaphor of wrestling that I have used in my title, I went to the story in Genesis about Jacob's emergence from his night of wrestling with the Angel of God, scathed but triumphant: "For I have seen God face to face, and my life is preserved."

As I wrote the book I came to see that it was a wrestling not with the disease alone, nor with the doctors and their medications and interventions, nor even with the "spite of Fortune." It was with the unfathomable mysteries, with Jacob's angel, with the dark man who came in the night and stayed and left—the angel at once of death and life—the Angel of God.

Since this is an intimate book, several persons close to me have been involved in its history. I am lucky to have three sons whose work has impinged closely upon its central theme. My doctor son is Adam Lerner, now an oncology fellow at Harvard's Dana Farber Cancer Institute. My ecologist and journalist son, Stephen Lerner, currently working out of Washington, has joined in watching over me at critical junctures, both personally and professionally. My son Michael Lerner, president of Commonweal, a health institute at Bolinas, California, has worked productively with an integral approach to cancer therapies, especially the "alternative" ones. I have profited from lively, sustained, and ongoing conversations with all three and from their contributions and criticisms.

My wife, Genevieve Edna Lerner, has shown courage and strength in coping with the course of my illness amidst her own crowded life. But for her the manuscripts would have come into the world laden with more of my crotchety excesses than have survived her astringent editorial skills. I owe more than I dare acknowledge to Evelyn Irsay, who had the forethought to spend some years working with a medical group before she became my personal assistant. Her experience and empathy have counted for much. I also consider myself lucky to have had Carol Houck Smith contributing her sensitive insights as editor.

ADDITIONAL NOTE TO THE READER

I have many readers and reviewers to thank for their generous response which made this new and more accessible edition possible. An author who commits a narrative of his own illness, one which is often critical of doctors and their role of authority, has to feel good to have it pass the exacting muster of reviewers who are physicians of the caliber of Jerome Groopman, Jay Meltzer, Siegfried Kra, and Gerald Weissman. Note that my themes reach beyond traditional clinical medicine to the mind/body connection and the centrality of the patient in the complex doctor/patient relation. Hence the generosity of these reviewers redeems my hope for the younger men and women who form the cutting edge of the medical profession today.

I add several updating notes. At eighty-eight, a decade after the onset of my lymphoma cancer, I can report that it remains well contained. As for my prostate cancer I still rejoice at rejecting the traditional choice between surgery and estrogen, and opting for the ministration of a then-experimental hormone which could avoid the trauma of both. Didn't all three (one medical reviewer asked) have the same chemical end result?

Perhaps. But what counted for me, beyond chemistry, even beyond psychology, was the end result for the total functioning organism and my deep inner sense of it.

My cardiac episode ("Thank God It's Only a Heart Attack!") also needs a somewhat acerbic update. In the summer of 1990, six years after the heart attack, I was hospitalized several times—needlessly, I now feel—for illusory symptoms that never got very far. The diagnosis was that some of my smaller arteries had clogged or closed.

Then unhappily I committed the further blunder of overextending myself—and my heart—in some seminars I gave in Washington. It led to another heart attack and a blocked major artery. I am now having to deal ruefully with the results, and to curb any future work excesses of mine.

At the same time I have been working with Dr. Dean Ornish, whose research on "reversing" heart problems (see p. 129) has become a wise and helpful book. Under his guidance I have re-embraced my earlier program of stress reduction and walking, and added a vegetarian diet. In doing so I have retrieved the patient's central role of taking charge of my discontents, and refreshed the hard-won principles I had reached after the three ordeals recounted here.

I dedicated the book to my daughter, Pamela Schofield, who died too young of a cancer. I add a memorial word for two close friends who struggled valiantly with their cancers and failed to survive them—Paul Cowan and Carmen Namuth. I am sad that they never got to read the pages that were in part written for them.

Anatole Broyard did read the book, in galleys, shortly before his own death from prostate cancer. His imaginative appreciation of it (in an overview piece on illness narratives) has inspirited me. His last essay for the *New York Times,* "Doctor, Talk to Me," will survive as a classic plea for the kind of communication that is all too rare.

Norman Cousins drank delight of battle for his "healing heart" over many years. In the end it proved a recalcitrant heart that outwitted his vigilance. Yet while he fought, his infectious writing reached and instructed an entire generation. He is remembered beyond friendship.

Just recently, with some pleasure, I stumbled on a comment I had missed earlier about Jacob's story in *Exodus,* of his wrestling with the angel of God. It came in a 1977 "self-interview" by the gifted American novelist, Walker Percy, who died of cancer in 1990: "I don't see why anyone should settle for anything less than Jacob, who actually grabbed aholt of God and wouldn't let go until God identified himself and blessed him."

After my more recent problems with my heart this has an even deeper meaning for me. I address this new edition to all who are determined to "grab aholt of God" and not let go, whether for dear life or dear death.

—M. L.

... And Jacob was left alone, and there wrestled a man with him until the breaking of the day. And when he saw that he prevailed not against him, he touched the bottom of his thigh; and the hollow of Jacob's thigh was out of joint as he wrestled with him. ... And Jacob called ... the place Peniel, "for I have seen God face to face, and my life is preserved."

— Gen. 32:24–30

I've made a long journey and been to a strange country, and I've seen the dark man very close.

— Thomas Wolfe, from the last letter he wrote

1. Contingency Is King

For the thing that I greatly feared is come upon me.

—Job

If I wrote a book called, "The World as I Found It," I should have to include a report on my body.

—Ludwig Wittgenstein, *Tractatus*

THIS IS ONE MAN'S JOURNEY away from death, toward life. It is at once a narrative of a cluster of illnesses and a meditation on them. There are many reasons a man gives himself for writing a memoir about an illness: his friends have egged him on; he wants to reach other sufferers; he thinks his example may do something to change the climate within which life-threatening illnesses are treated. There is a kernel of truth for me in each. Yet my real reason is an experiential one. I passed through a searing experience that tested and changed me in ways I never foresaw. And like the Ancient Mariner I want to tell my story, to whatever listeners it finds.

The austere medical scientists call this kind of evidence "anecdotal," as distinguished from the rigorously "experimental," where you have "populations" being studied statistically along with their "control groups." I don't mind the designation but suggest that the "narrative" mode is better. It is a term emerging in literary criticism which has spread to other human disciplines as a legitimate method of getting at some essential truths.

I add that the ultimate experiment is life itself. It was Emerson who had the acumen to observe that "wherever you touch life, it bleeds." He furnished no statistics.

When we get the news it tells us that "in the Midst of Life We Are in Death." I call it the news because it comes abruptly, this dread, fateful message, and it comes not by any design you can fathom but by the misshapen perversity of chance. The messenger is the doctor, and when the news is bad its molten associations fix themselves forever in the memory.

How many have heard the news, in how many diverse settings! Senator Paul Tsongas of Massachusetts, retiring from public life in his forties, told an interviewer in 1984 that his doctor's brief words, "You have lymphoma," were the most terrifying he had heard in his life. An editor friend of mine in

Los Angeles got a call from her internist. "I have dreadful, dreadful news for you" was how he began. He may have meant to prepare her for the shock. He couldn't have been more brutal.

Almost always there is the sense of being singled out by some evil chance. In the territory of the ill, contingency is king. His kingdom, as seen by his subjects, seems riddled with the irrational, full of omens and portents, ready for the irruption of any capricious event—side effects from medications, malady generating malady, symptoms and counter-symptoms, sleeplessness, hopelessness, and always the dread pain. I was to learn all too well the ways of this wayward contingency, wayward not only in whom it strikes but where and how, and who survives and on what terms.

In my case the news came when I was intensely involved with life. After a quarter-century at Brandeis University I had left my American Civilization chair at seventy and begun another career, teaching the behavioral sciences at a graduate school in California. I led a bicoastal life, commuting biweekly between New York City (where I lived with my wife Jenny) and my teaching at San Diego, Irvine, and Los Angeles. I wrote a syndicated column as a self-appointed civilization watcher, had done a dozen books over a forty-year span, had seen something of the world. There were five grown children and eight grandchildren, and I was fiercely involved with them.

In its restless passion for power, experience, and innovation, twentieth-century America was deeply Faustian, and in my own restless questings and hungers I shared much of it. The resulting hubris, which tempted the gods, was there in full measure. My journals at the time reflect a euphoria which had a compulsive quality. "Life is good," said one of my diary notes in 1977. It was a steady refrain in my conversations with my family and students. I liked Rilke's reported last words, "Never forget, children, life can be beautiful". My own verb was more assertive: not *can be* but *is.*

To give some context to the news when it came, let me note that my seventies were years still full of travel, classes, lecturing, writing. I had done some long TV interviews, sat for a profile of myself in *People* magazine, written a book on the Kennedys which was timed to Ted's ill-fated presidential campaign. I caught planes, flagged taxis, wrote last-minute notes on planes for my talks, got to my destinations. I acted as if there were to be an endless succession of such days. I saw my world and its life force as an inexhaustible treasure trove, and almost fancied myself immortal. The ground I walked on was the familiar ground of my life—firm, tangible. The solid earth held, or seemed to.

Thus when the first rumblings of trouble came, it was of trouble in my paradise. Somewhere around 1977 I developed a prostate problem, and after a ravaging biopsy (there were to be three in all), the pathology results were happily negative. I got word of them after a seminar at San Diego and celebrated at lunch with a group of students. It was my first brush with the theme of cancer.

Whatever the prostate problem was, surfacing and getting attention, there was—beneath the surface—an intermittent sense of cramp and pain that brought some discomfort. It continued through 1979 and 1980, into 1981, and evoked an anxiety I tried to deny.

I have to add that at one point there was an episode of intense emotional stress that made life somewhat rockier than I was prepared to admit. Yet I find some characteristic journal notations by December 1980, when I was to turn seventy-eight: "I am alive and well and will have another decade or more." A week earlier I had written, "I shall triumph." Clearly I was troubled enough to be trying to reassure myself.

A measure of reassurance came in January 1981, when John Van Doorn asked me to do a cover piece on aging for his new magazine, *Next,* which focused on futures. It was a pretty swaggering piece that spilled over into the boastful, expressing a too triumphant sense of having reached my late seventies still functional. I called it "The Delights of Aging." The picture John ran with it displayed me against a barn door in California, lifting a long exercise bar high above my head, like one of those strongmen in the workout ads. It was an idiotic thing to do, this display of exhibitionism. I see it now as marking the high point of my illusory Eden, before the Fall.

Just how fast I was running became clear when my publishers sent me on the usual promotion trip for the Kennedy book. A mystery pain plagued me in Boston and Washington, but in Chicago for some reason it gave me a respite. I recall gazing at the Chicago highrise skyline from my hotel window at sunset, experiencing an epiphany of reborn assurance that it had all been a passing malady and that triumph lay ahead.

It didn't. What lay ahead was more intense pain. It started in earnest the third week of January 1981, when my journal noted my broken nights and my sleepy afternoons, adding, "But I shall ride my luck." This was followed by "another scary spell" for four nights, and a weight loss of five pounds. My journal suspected "a cancer somewhere in my gut."

My long-time internist, Jeremiah Barondess, arranged a barium test and an abdominal scan. This meant missing my California classes and giving up the teaching quarter, which added an element of depression to my mystery pains.

Jerry and I were good friends as well as doctor-and-patient. He was a seasoned diagnostician of the first rank, with a witty, astringent style, a literary flair, and an analytical sharpness. At first, offering some hope, he talked of an abdominal "obstruction," but when he summoned me after the scans I could sense clearly enough that the news was not good.

"My boy," he began (he was more than twenty years my junior), "you have a problem." The tests showed a greatly en-larged spleen, "probably a carcinoma." The prognosis? That depended on the kind of tumor I had (if indeed I had one), and where it was, and how advanced or recent, and how treatable. There had been some therapeutic progress in certain kinds of tumors. My age was a factor but not decisive. Whatever the site, he added, there would probably have to be chemotherapy and/ or radiation. "Right now we have to get you to the hospital."

I felt the shock deep in my offending gut. Suddenly I had lost my center of gravity, which depended on my belief in my body as a given, a habitation for my "self." The universe which had sustained me for my seventy-eight years dissolved in a single swift stroke. And I knew I should somehow have to put to-gether a new universe.

Breaking my story, and taking a jump of more than a year, I have to add something I didn't know at the start: that in a serious illness the news comes in installments, and the second may make the initial news look pale. The first installment told me I "had a problem," as my internist put it, as gently as he could. The second told me how much time I had left.

It came when everything seemed to be going downhill, and I was scared, and wanted someone with big authority to tell me where I stood. So Jerry Barondess called in a distinguished lymphoma specialist for consultation. My wife Jenny and I came to see him in an examining room at his hospital. He was sympathetic, took my history carefully, sorted through the re-ports on the pathology of the tumor, listened and thumped, and seemed saddened by what he found. It took scarcely a half hour, and he was about to dismiss me with some formula words which, however ambiguous, betrayed that mine was a forlorn case.

But I didn't mean to be fobbed off. So I pressed him: What was the prognosis and what were my chances? I was under the right care, he said, but my large-cell lymphoma, always a difficult type, was in an advanced state. The chemotherapy I had, which included Adriamycin and Cytoxan, was ordinarily adequate, but he felt I needed something more "aggressive," and probably radiation as well. My age was against me. At seventy-nine my statistical chances were not good.

I pressed him again: How bad? Finally I got out of him the harsh truth, this time the unvarnished "news." "I should guess," he said as kindly as he could, "that you don't have much more than six months." In the cab home Jenny and I sat very close.

It was a turning point for me. I had been a man of words, accustomed to orient myself in terms of the territory of ideas. But here I was, alone with my cancer, ignorant of its grammar, syntax, and vocabulary, of its chemistry and biology, of the dynamics of its growth and treatment, of the physics of its acceleration and the statistics of my mortality. I had to rely on the experts who understood these things. But after the reeling news I decided to fight back, if only to show that, however ravaged by the dividing cell, I was not a statistic but a sovereign person.

I had all along suspected that my lymphoma was serious, but until this consultation with one of the authorities in the field no one had quantified so sharply my prospects for survival.

It was a rough awakening, but a chastening one. It taught me to rally every resource, to assert my will not only to survive but to function as fully as I could, perhaps to prevail.

In our time we are coming to understand that none of us is immune from the necessity of facing—at one or another point in our histories—some life-threatening episode. Cancers, strokes, heart ailments, Parkinson's, Alzheimer's, multiple sclerosis, AIDS—the diseases that beset us are varied, and their treatment has been the subject of intensive, experimental study. Now, increasingly, the responses of the patients to their ailments are capturing attention in and out of the medical profession. In a curious sense medical advances, even as they have heightened expectations, have not lessened anxieties; as hope has risen, the fear of missing out becomes sharper. And the pale rider on his pale horse becomes all the more the apparition to overcome.

How to overcome him became my obsession. The answer took time to shape itself. If it was to be a combat then I had to engage it with everything I had—knowledge and guile, ways covert as well as overt, outwaiting and outwitting the enemy. I still didn't know what resources I could muster, or with what authority to take charge when the medical judgments I got were in conflict.

But I have run ahead of my narrative in order to get to what I now see as the defining event. By presenting me with the ultimate "news," my encounter with the lymphoma specialist, in that narrow examining room, taught me that the war ahead was real and brought the enemy home to me.

2. The Locus of the Evil

We say we die of some particular disease, but we don't. We die from the whole life we have lived.

— Charles Peguy

Life can only be understood backwards, but it must be lived forwards.

— Sören Kierkegaard

Every man bears his death within himself, as the fruit bears its stone.

— Rainer Maria Rilke

I RETURN NOW TO the weeks that followed my admission to New York Hospital. The hospital stay was the first step in Jerry Barondess's campaign to root out my disease at the source. I entered the hospital reluctantly—but I entered. My few previous hospital episodes had not predisposed me to take kindly to the hospital experience. I know that hospitals are necessary. I have been in some of the best, in which I include the one I entered. I know the effort that doctors, nurses, and attendants have taken to humanize the usual severity of the hospital environment. But I never fully understood until then that the beginnings of healing must be the restoration of the selfhood which the dire news had all but shattered. Nor had I understood as sharply as I do now how completely a patient is expected to surrender selfhood to the doctors and to the apparatus of a hospital.

It was an environment that ended whatever controls I had exercised over my prehospital life. Instead, the controls were taken over by a highly structured, artificial hospital society, with mechanized schedules and a dreary, sanitized ambiance. As with every institution where rules and discipline must be enforced and often grow rigid, the needs of the institutional process tend to crowd out the needs of the patient.

There was something else that carried over from my past hospital experience: the apprehension of the unknown thing that could happen, once I passed through the reception, got my wrist tag, was allotted my room and unpacked my bag. A nurse misreading her instructions, an infected needle, interns or residents still learning their way, a doctor's blundering judgment, a surgeon's unresourceful decision, a stray bacillus or other organism finding its way through the fertile hospital environment to my own organism—these were not imaginings but attested facts of life in the medical jungle.

I have to confess that I had been soured, during an earlier

hospital stay, by a bleak, adversarial book on medical practices, *Medical Nemesis*, by Ivan Illich. It was a depressing book to take along on a hospital jaunt, for it was an unsparing challenge to the underlying assumptions of the thinking on medical institutions. It presented an abrasive analysis of the doctor-induced ("iatrogenic") diseases you may get in the course of coping with the one you brought to the hospital.

By itself this would not have troubled me overmuch, since I am bullish rather than bilious by disposition. What did trouble me was the linkage of these accidental factors with my prevailing sense of an environment over which I had no control.

Whatever my skepticism, I felt we had dawdled away too much time. My overriding need was to take hold of this tumor and wrench its neck—however anatomically wrong my metaphor was. Getting at its source and nature could only be done in a hospital, where I would have my first sustained introduction to the sequence of hospital tests that forms the medical base for treating a major illness.

The prevailing medical paradigm rests on the proposition that the patient somewhere houses the key to his malady and treatment, that it is something material which can be put under a lens (or into a computer) and studied, decoded, interpreted. In its economy of method, medicine tries all lesser interventions before resorting to major ones. I recalled a conversation with Jerry Barondess on the occasion of an earlier hospital stay, in May 1976, when he explained the Barondess Unified Field Theory of Internal Medicine to me: "It's quite simple," he said. "What to do is measurably clearer than what's the matter." That was what the tests were about—man stretching his ingenuity to get beneath and beyond the skin into the inside of a patient's body, reaching to the desired area or organ while leaving the organism relatively intact.

Reaching not just to get a picture. Medicine has done wonders in photographing every human crevice. Nothing escapes it. But you can't take a picture apart and play with its chemical ingredients. The ultimate object was to get at the thing itself, however minute, which would reveal under the intense scrutiny of pathologists the source of the evil.

Since I contained the evil, I was the locus of the search. At the time I wasn't this metaphysical about it. I was too busy being explored. I was wheeled everywhere for "procedures," which I came to define as anything whose intrusion and torture fell short of cutting me open in a major way. Every aperture that might debouche on the desired booty was explored. They even sent me, by an underground tunnel, to Memorial Hospital across the avenue, where an inventive young specialist had devised a way of puncturing me above the spleen and inserting a tube through which he could try to snip off tissue enough to examine. The procedure was ingenious but it didn't work.

Despite the resourcefulness of these explorations nothing worked. It took weeks. I was exasperated with this evasive tissue of mine. How arrogant of it to elude the best medical technology of our time! Yet I had a sneaking pride that in the vast arena of statistical precision my organism became a statistic they couldn't take for granted.

In the end there was nothing left except the plan to open me up surgically, extract the tissue for study, and—while they were about it—lift out my offending spleen. I was dismayed. I prided myself on being a functionalist. Was there, I asked, no *function* that the spleen performed? To believe that there was indeed none seemed to cast doubt upon the prudence of God or the tenets of evolution, or both.

I had a conference with the senior surgeon, Dr. William Barnes, who wore the mantle of experience reassuringly. I was not to worry. The spleen was useful as part of the immune system (if so it was a defender who had defected to the enemy!) but the body could get along without it. I tried to think of three spleenless people I knew, failed, and gave up on my preliminary skirmish with the authorities, who swept away objections from an ornery old man who clearly knew little about anatomy or physiology.

On that score they were right enough. But whatever my medical ignorance, I trusted my intuitive sense of my own organism. Instead of fearing I would be losing an essential organ I came instead to feel I would be ridding my organism of a heavy cancerous one. So I went along with them, relieved that I could strike at the Adversary who had made the blunder of concentrating his forces where they were encapsulated and could be captured.

But could they? When I emerged from a morning of surgery and intensive care, the first thing they told me was that the operation had gone well—but that I still had the spleen. For Dr. Barnes, on getting to the swollen organ, found it so entangled with other organs that it couldn't be lifted out with the necessary surgical precision.

I can describe my mood best by quoting from a journal entry written on the evening after the surgery in the well-nigh illegible scrawl of a very shaky hand:

> *February 15, 1981*   God be thanked! But alas, the spleen is still in me. Barnes and Co. couldn't get it out. Highly emotional day. Monday night in hospital I worked hard on column "Does American Civilization Have a Future?" (Strange topic to be doing.) Very high when I did it. . . . Ah well, the spleen still there. Will have to be shrunk by the same chemotherapy and/or radiation. . . . But here I still am, propped up

in bed. . . . Dreaming dreams that seem remarkably
real until I wake. . . . The eternal ones of the dream.
Who are they?

Who indeed? My dreams have always been vivid and multiple. Over many years I feel I have dreamed most of the classical
dreams and perhaps the romantic and surrealist ones, too. I
have fancied myself a connoisseur of dreams, trying to capture
and digest them immediately on waking, before they dissolve.
Dreams form for me one of the ultimate mysteries, like love,
God, chance, and death.

Sleep in hospitals is at best intermittent, broken by "procedures," tests, and schedules, and dreams are often transformed
by pain and drugs into hypnogogic states, between sleep and
waking. The result for me was that the dividing line between
reality and imagining got blurred, and I spent much of my time
in a haze.

Even when writing my columns—three a week then—I did
so in the shadowy, drugged, half-world on the edge of the unconscious. I kept telling myself that this was exactly how Coleridge and DeQuincy wrote in their opium-induced ecstasy. It
didn't produce any masterpieces for me, yet, going back to my
scrawls, they seem to have profited from the touch of the manic
and from tapping the shadowy realm of my unconscious.

As a high school boy in New Haven I had picked up stray
remaindered copies of the journals of Emerson, Thoreau, and
Pepys, and I dreamed of keeping one myself and having some
events in my life worthy of being entered in it. Much later, as a
young editor in New York's swirling life, I started a journal and
have kept it discontinuously ever since. I was drawn to it first as
a mode of self-vigilance and self-discovery. But it also became
fun—a repository of notions for writings to come, an arena for

fighting out emotional and intellectual battles and keeping track of the vagaries of selfhood.

So I turned to it in the hospital, to have some record of the jumbled memories of those initial weeks and months of crisis. For the same reason I kept working on columns and book projects, as continuity with the underground current of my life which the news of the cancer had broken.

The greatest threat anyone with a radical illness runs is the threat to the continuity of selfhood. If that gets shattered there is nothing to fight back with. The doctors, nurses and orderlies, testers and counters, report writers, sometimes even friends and family, see the patient as someone being acted on: "Patch him up and get him out." The patient alone can fight that perception by an active perception of self. My writing and journals were signals I sent myself that under it all the major current of my life was still flowing. It was the best therapy I could muster.

A mortally sick person suffers repeatedly from a communication crisis. The only people who can tell him what is happening objectively are in the business of arresting and postponing his death. They are not in the business of communicating much to him, and in my experience rarely is it the whole truth at all times. This applies especially in a diagnostic crisis when the authorities themselves don't yet know the truth and don't want to frighten the patient.

When Dr. Barnes got to the spleen and couldn't remove it he snipped off a bit of suspicious tissue attached to the pancreas, perhaps riding it (I fancied) like a hitchhiker. He reported the event to Jerry, but neither of them told me. Cancer of the pancreas is even more dangerous than large-cell lymphoma, however advanced. The chances of my survival, in that case, would have been even slimmer than they were. Until they were certain, they decided as experienced doctors to keep the news from me.

Yet I did learn about this new entrant in my drama. There was a hospital team of interns and residents who made their rounds of visits every morning with the regularity of the postman. One of them was a remarkably able fourth-year medical student. We hit it off and had long talks, more candid than any with my doctors. He reminded me of students at Williams and Brandeis with whom I had broken through the conventional academic stiffness and from whom I had learned much.

Before the surgery he had detailed, for my edification, the nature and ways of the spleen. Now he told me, reluctantly, about the tissue found on the pancreas, and as gently as he could he related what was known about cancer of the pancreas. I had some bad days and nights, when I tossed about in bed with my new knowledge. Yet I am indebted to him for assuming that this man, weighted with years, could take whatever life brought.

I told Jerry Barondess that I knew, and he might have been relieved. Did he know all along that the student told me? Or was he, like my wife Jenny, annoyed at the well-meant elaborations by friendly, voluble students? Jerry never volunteered it, either way. But several days later I got a call from him. He was laconic and witty as always. "I have good news for you." he said. "They have finished the pathology of the tissue. The good news is that you have lymphoma."

Contingency again but good contingency. Machiavelli gave the name *Fortuna* to the goddess of Chance, as against *Necessità,* which marked the givens that couldn't be changed. Now in her wild gyrations the goddess swirled in my direction.

The question for the doctors all along was whether the tumor was simply sitting *on* the pancreas as a place to alight, like a boll weevil on a cotton stalk, or whether it was in fact a cancer *of* the pancreas. They hadn't wanted to tell me about it until they knew the answer.

In one sense they were right. It is a gray area in decision making, a question perhaps less in medicine than in moral philosophy. They didn't want to plow me up needlessly when I required all my mental strength for recovery from the severe surgery, and from the disappointment at waking to find my spleen still there. They must have felt it was not a court proceeding where the whole truth was required.

But was I right too? I was neither an adolescent nor mentally fragile but a grown man, a quarter-century older than any of them. What I required was their candor, otherwise their authority was shaken.

In our several moral philosophies our difference of viewpoint derived from something still deeper, the respective paradigms we had of the doctor–patient relationship. In their paradigm the doctor was at the center of the entire cluster of relationships, and the patient was only one member—even if the crucial one—of the cluster that radiated from the doctor. In the paradigm I was just starting to shape, the patient took the doctor's place at the center, and the rest radiated from him.

Looking back now I feel it turns on whether a doctor knows something for certain. If not, he can use his judgment, as Jerry did. If he does know, he should tell it. I may be expressing only a deeply American moral dilemma. The Japanese doctors didn't tell even their Emperor Hirohito, with all his divinity, that he had a terminal intestinal cancer. There are many beasts lurking in this jungle.

An excerpt from my journal at the hospital:

March 2, 1981 I shall live, and have a chance to get well. Which is what counts. I have now known it for five days, since Friday noon, when Jerry called to tell

me it was lymphoma after all, not a cancer of the
pancreas as Barnes and he had both suspected. This
has been a terrible month in my life—the worst since
Pam's death.

The 2 or 3 days after the surgery, when I didn't
know whether it might be cancer *of* the pancreas, not
just *on* it, were hellish days. Jenny and I felt bleak. I
think she almost gave up. I suspect I did. I couldn't
face it—not the death only but the manner of it, without having much chance really to fight. . . . Those who
spoke with me then knew how sunk I was in despond.

Yet I did confront the near certainty of death if the
diagnosis should turn out that way. And I was re-
signed in the sense that I have had a good life and a
long one—and if God felt it should end now—that
was it. . . .

I remember the phone call from Jerry, Friday noon,
bearing the "good news" (!) of lymphoma. . . . I called
Steve immediately and he told Mike, then later Adam
arrived. I was terribly weak, all wired, in pain, hardly
able to move. Yet there was joy in my heart! . . .

The days since have been up and down, but the
tubes are out, and I have shit twice and am getting
ready for a third, and hope to resolve the problem of
the pain in the night, and am waiting to gain some
strength. The A.M. today was crummy and sleepy (co-
deine last night) but I *did* write a whole column after
lunch, had a half-dozen phone conversations, walked
the corridor with Jen. I just turned back (in this journal) to William James on overdrawing one's "moral
drawing account." I overdrew my energy account and
incurred a *hubris.*

3. The Torment of Choice

Life is short, and Art long, the crisis fleeting, experience perilous, and decision difficult.

— Hippocrates, *Aphorisms*

A will which resolves on nothing is no actual will; a characterless man never reaches a decision.

— G.W.F. Hegel, *Philosophy of Right*

I will show you how not to be a dead man in life.

— D. H. Lawrence

Choice would hardly be significant if it did not take effect in outward action, and if it did not, when expressed in deeds, make a difference in things.

— John Dewey, *Philosophies of Freedom*

S O WE HAD LEARNED the nature of the beast and laid bare his origin. But how to overcome him? In the grim progression of tasks in medicine, the problem of treatment carries with it the thorny question of choice.

For a patient to make final choices in the domain of illness, where the doctor's authority is sovereign, is a form of *lèse majesté*. Although I had made some forays into rebellion in past medical episodes, I knew I couldn't play Jefferson and write my own Declaration of Independence. The difference was that Jefferson felt he had "Nature and Nature's God" on his side, while in my case the doctors had preempted the forces of Nature, speaking for its laws, and had become gods in their own right.

While railing at this, what I faced was a course of chemotherapy to overcome the spreading of the hostile cells and to kill every last one of them. I had heard enough about chemotherapy to respect and fear its effects, but my assessment was not rooted in knowledge. I knew the theory—that the researchers had experimentally found some combination of chemicals which the doctors poured into the organism against the killer cells they were intended in turn to kill. But if I was to believe in these chemicals it would have to be not by knowledge but by a leap of faith, which I was unprepared to take.

There were other problems of choice as well. Everyone stricken with some "dread" disease must at some point confront the question of how much to talk about it, and how much to reveal.

Understandably there is the smell of taboo around life-threatening maladies, since a society tribally tries to protect its integrity and sees a stricken person as a threat to the well-being of all. Very early, and throughout my illness, I tried to be honest about my cancer, with myself and others. I paid a price for my openness. As word spread, my lecture requests and magazine assignments melted away. Max Lerner healthy in his late seven-

ties presented quite a different image from Max Lerner with
cancer—and God knows what else—on his way out of life's
arena. We immure our sick in hospitals but we also invent ingenious ways of moving them offstage, banishing them from life's
center, making their healing and self-healing more difficult.

I came to understand early that there is no place to hide and
no point in hiding. The reality had to be faced, but how to define
it? We don't know what health is until we fall ill and lose it.
Like many who get seriously sick I saw health as the absence of
illness, just as we see illness as the absence of health—which is
question-begging, since it defines each in terms of the other.
They are both, of course, polar aspects of a basic state of the
organism.

I had to form some idea of the true nature of illness and
health. I sensed that their major components, the subjective
sense of self and the objective state of the organism, are both
deep within our consciousness, each intricately linked with the
other. My subjective sense might lag behind the reality in a
depressive funk, or might seek to prod and cajole it into improv-
ing itself. But the two are never far from each other, tied in a
strange necessity that goes with the total organism.

From such a perspective health and illness are the double
signature of this necessity. In time I came to understand health
as a working equilibrium of the systems of the organism in a
functioning balance. From the same perspective, illness is in
turn a breaking of that equilibrium, destabilizing the balance of
the whole. Recovery is the achieving of a new equilibrium. I
was trying to understand, in functional terms, what had happened to me (illness), where I had been before (health), and
where I wanted to go (healing).

Part of my problem came out of my conditionings. I had
spent my life teaching and writing on politics and the human
disciplines, whose essence was the need for choice between al-

ternatives. In the early 1970s I had given workshops at the Esalen Institute, at Big Sur, California. More recently I had been
teaching seminars at a strongly humanistic Graduate School of
Human Behavior, at San Diego. In both settings my students
and I had to explore the sovereign mind and its capacity to
create its environment by choices. Now I was, in effect, being
instructed to forgo choices because there were only technical
ones and surrender my mind and organism to the custody of the
medical deities.

It is time to introduce my family. Except in recent work on
family systems therapy, the medical model tends to scant the
role of the family in illness and healing. Yet nothing is more
critical to the human ecology of a dangerous illness. In Tol-
stoyan terms ours was a happy family, performing well the two
functions a family has in such situations: to act as the sheath of
caring for its sick members, and to serve as context for the
patient's decision making.

My family, broadly supportive, was divided on the issue of
choices. My wife, Jenny, spent decades as a clinical psycholo-
gist at Payne Whitney Clinic, in the Cornell medical complex of
which New York Hospital formed part. She had been the ador-
ing daughter of a surgeon and had inherited his strong reality
sense. She had been my student at Sarah Lawrence but had
pretty positive judgments of her own. Although believing in the
role of the mind in maintaining health, she thought my early
California adventurism of will therapies was mostly arrant ten-
dermindedness.

Our youngest son, Adam, then in his junior year at Yale
Medical School, was hard-wire in his approach but tolerant
enough of my doubts to engage me in delightful philosophical
discussions of the organism and its laws. Later he was to decide
to do his residency in oncology, and he is presently a fellow in

oncology at Dana Farber Institute, at Harvard.

Of my other two sons, Stephen has all along been a strong environmentalist. At the time of my illness, working with his brother Michael in California, he focused on the effects of industrial pollutants on health. He later came East, to New York and Washington, as a journalist and penologist, involved especially with the young in foster home and prison environments. He brought the quizzical, lucid eye of a practiced ecologist to my succession of difficulties.

My oldest son, Michael, was especially caught up in my case history. He had left the Yale political theory faculty and founded Commonweal, a community where he worked with chronically ill adults, pioneering a program of self-understanding and self-healing for them, with a blend of nutrition, meditation, stress avoidance, and a favoring environment. Michael was moved, in part by my illness, to probe more deeply into cancer. He has been leading a series of "retreats" for cancer patients, to help them deal affirmatively with their illness and their attitudes toward it, and has completed a book, *The Geography of Hope,* on the choices a patient can make in available cancer therapies.

My two daughters, both older than their brothers, were less professionally involved in my illness but, with their families, no less supportive of me. The younger, Joanna Townsend, then in London, now in New York and Dallas, brought an earthy quality of realism that I sorely needed during my torment of choice. Constance Russell, my first-born, ran a religious-psychological support group in San Diego, and we discussed love, God, and health by letter and talk. I add my two sisters—Sylvia Williams and Ida Borish, four and six years my elders, both in Fort Lauderdale, Florida—who continued in the close-knit familial tradition which our early immigrant origins had bred into us.

It was a far-flung but strongly cohesive clan. It offers an

instance of how deeply a family with close ties can be affected, in its direction, by the illness of one of its members. But much of this came later. At the time it was a polar struggle for me, and my doctors and Michael were the two poles, the first with their built-in commitment to traditional treatment, the other with his strong inclination toward "integral" health care.

While my immediate impulse was away from the chemotherapy and the radiation that might follow, I was—as so many cancer patients are today—in a crisis of belief. I had strong doubts about the bruising effects of medical technology in these extreme illnesses, yet I could not get myself to embrace the still dubious alternative treatment wholeheartedly. So there I was, a self-tormented creature, doubting while I strained to believe, caught between a medical world that was suffering sharp challenge and one that had not yet come to birth.

A bit of personal history may shed some light on the two forces that tugged at me. Man, as Shakespeare had it, is only "a poor forked creature with a head fantastically carved." Yet each of us travels an intellectual and emotional life journey, shaped in part by the turf we inhabit and the climate of ideas that envelops us.

My home was in New York, where I had spent a half-century since my first job after graduate school. I was tossing about on a hospital bed in that "mischievous and marvelous" city, to use E. B. White's phrase, wrestling with my choices. I was a child of New York and of its fierce intellectual rationalism which made it the world's cultural capital. But I had also embraced selective elements of the Californian subculture which wanted to start everything anew.

In my workshops and seminars there, through the late 1960s and the 1970s, I touched on disciplines in the antechamber of what was becoming "behavioral," or "holistic," medicine. Implicit in this phase of my thinking was the idea that in the realm of the human organism—as indeed in the conduct of life—the sense of the possible, fueled by the power of the imagination and will, plays a formative role.

Thus, as the bicoastal child of one strain of thought and the stepchild of another that challenged it, I felt there were two selves engaged within me, making conflicting claims upon my decisions.

This was the stream of my thinking when the cancer news and the need to choose a treatment broke into it. I insert all this as context, when so many involved with illness and its healing forget context. They stress symptoms, diagnosis, treatment, without imbedding all three in the intellectual and spiritual life history of the patient. We don't die from some particular disease, wrote the French thinker Charles Peguy, but "from the whole life we have lived." I came to know from my experience that the source of my illness was my entire life. But as it turned out, so was the source of my healing.

Jerry Barondess brought in Dr. Richard Silver, who headed hematology-oncology (blood and cancer) at New York Hospital. I liked him. I knew that the great specialized cancer hospital was the one across the street—Sloan-Kettering Memorial Hospital. While both hospitals used the same philosophy, Memorial was known world-wide for its specialized staff and research. Yet I didn't shift to it, feeling that my doctors would give me the skill and extra attention a patient in chemotherapy needs—if indeed I decided to take it on.

I resisted deciding too quickly. Michael and I talked much about it. Even before the cancer struck he had suggested slowing down the urgencies of my daily life. He didn't push it now, saying I had to follow my deepest bent. But I knew that his own preference was to stress the quality of life that went with the choices. He made it clear that radical chemotherapy, both in its course and consequences, was bound to be drastic, especially at my age. I sensed that he inclined toward a gentler alternative discipline, even while he felt that no one else could make that decision for me.

I could no longer ignore the fact of my two warring selves. I knew that if I went in for a punishing round of chemotherapy—and perhaps a round of radiation afterward—it would be an anguished experience both for my organism and for the quality of my life. I also knew that if we failed to deal decisively with that tumor in my gut, the result would be even worse: death itself.

I was caught between two savagings, hence my torment of choice. My doctors were getting impatient with my dawdling. I didn't blame them. They had a chemotherapy protocol which Dick Silver explained to me: half the patients on cooperating hospital lists would be treated by one mixture of chemotherapy, the other half by another. I was somewhat put off by the chanciness of this: What if I got into the less effective half, even though both were meant to be broadly similar. "Without the protocol," as Adam told me later, "we would all be in deep muck." I agreed that it was not as bad as research with a placebo, but, as with all large-scale testing projects, the guinea pig element was there.

I didn't like the role, and at that juncture I was in no mood to be hurried. Each of the diverging roads could take me in an unknown direction with consequences I was too uninformed to calculate. While I thought of exploring several "alternative" treatment centers—the Livingston Clinic at San Diego and the Simonton Clinic at Houston—I didn't believe, deep down, that I would pass up the chemotherapy and opt for nontraditional treatment.

I felt, nevertheless, that for decisions to be made there had to be choices. Otherwise I was on a roller coaster to an unknown land. The tumult of choice was confusing, but the necessity of choice was none the less real. It was a self-discipline I had to traverse, that no gravely sick person can escape by placing it on the shoulders of others.

I needed time to think, not in this alien land called a hospital but at home, in my own chair, looking out over my river. So with the benevolent consent of Jerry Barondess (he was getting used to my ornery ways) I went home for a week. I meant to consult my innermost oracle, my sense of my organism. I recalled how often I had told my seminar students to "follow the organism." Now I was doing that.

4. The Universe of the Ill

He has seen but half the Universe who never has been shown the house of pain.

— Ralph Waldo Emerson

The universe of the ill is different from the universe of the well.

— Aldous Huxley, quoted by his doctor

Do you not see how necessary a world of pain and trouble is to school an intelligence and make it a soul?

— John Keats, *Letters*

There was in the world a pain concerning which God had set an example of pure and absolute silence.

— John Updike, *Bech Is Back*

YOU ENTER A HOSPITAL with the burden of your fears and hopes. You leave it with both still there but in a very different combination. That's why, if you sit watching at the reception office, the patients entering show a gray sameness of anxiety and depression. If you watch at the departure door the lucky ones seem to be emerging from a dark tunnel.

Jenny came and signed out for me and I went down in the traditional wheelchair to the hospital exit. These entries, exits and re-entries, which go with the territory of the ill, were to become a too familiar ritual in my succession of hospital surgeries and treatments.

I was shaky in the cab. I gazed at the normal world of cars and shopkeepers and young women wheeling their baby carriages, and lovers with their arms entwined, much as a newly released prisoner stares at the normal world from which he was cut off.

Home was bittersweet, sweet because it was our territory, Jenny's and mine, bitter because I didn't know when I would see it again. So I caressed the much read and loved books and gazed out of our windows at the East River tugboats pushing the ships and barges. The scene was a symbol for me of the stream of experience running through our lives. I found my favorite chair, savored the food, riffled through my mail and magazines, and felt for a fleeting moment in touch again with the universe of the well.

I clung to my ties with that universe. I was cancer-ridden, my weight had dropped sharply, and I got little reassurance from any mirror. The "I" that stared back at me was startlingly different from the "I" in the California photo, the one with my arms stretched to the sky, lifting the bars.

In most of our lives we take Time with a capital T for granted, but my illness left me with a sharp consciousness of its implacable brevity. I would take my chances on my cancer in a

timeless universe. In my present state I desperately wanted
Time to stand still.

It didn't. So I retraversed my choices and found little that
was new. Yet I did find one perspective that might clarify
things. It was the matter of irreversibility. The chemotherapy
might not work, but if I didn't try it now I would never know—
and later it might be too late. Without it, including all its nega-
tives, the tumor might grow with no redress. The hackneyed
adage was true after all: "Better safe than sorry!"

There wasn't the same urgency about the alternative, or "ad-
junctive," therapies. I could still use them to supplement the
chemotherapy but not the other way around. Moreover, I could
apply them myself. I wouldn't need a hospital for that. Wherever I found myself I could use my own affirmations.

Looking back at it from the safer haven of today, all this
seems pretty self-evident. But earlier it wasn't. I had to work it
out within myself but I did it more clearly in the quiet of my
home, seeking a larger frame and strategy, a wider knowing.

I was learning the arts of being ill. "If Contingency is King,"
I wrote later in my journal, "then in his Kingdom you have to
live from day to day at his will."

So after an easeful week at home I came back to the hospital
and started my protocol. The drug of choice—actually of non-
choice—assigned to me was Adriamycin, combined with
Cytoxan and two other drugs. I got weighed and measured so
that Dr. Silver could calculate how much to give me. Too little
and the killer cells would gain on me, too much and it would
savage my system. The doctor administering it had to become a
master of equilibration. Fortunately for me, as Jerry had known
in choosing him, Dick Silver had exactly the right quality of
concentration on the individual case.

That the power to heal and the power to kill are often combined is a paradox that goes deep to the nature of things. In the anthropology of medicine we know that the primitive medicine man had control over charms and poisons together. In Elizabethan England the apothecary and chemist were the only physicians available to most. Modern chemotherapy builds on basic nineteenth- and twentieth-century research, which made biochemistry the heart of our pharmacological armory. As literary associations rumbled through my mind I found it ironic that someone who had all but flunked chemistry should be staking his life on the proposition that a mixture of chemical molecules was possessed of the potency to kill the killer cells before they killed him.

It was a wager in its purest form, not on the fights or horses but on life itself. The celebrator of Broadway sporting life, Damon Runyan, calculated that "all life is six-to-five against." It was meant cynically, but I would have gladly settled for the odds. I gathered that in my coming chemical wager, despite my being bolstered by the weight of modern medical technology, the odds were more steeply against me.

I had been much taken by Tennyson's *Idylls of the King.* I now half expected Merlin, maguslike, to enter with the cup. If I was to drink the healing potion I should have liked it in a silver chalice, preceded by a flourish of trumpets. Instead there came a very businesslike nurse pushing a trolley mounted with a large inverted bottle. I didn't drink the potion, which was fed into my system intravenously through a needle inserted in my wrist. Lying in bed I used to watch the clockwork drip-drip of the liquid which slowly, efficiently—along with my other drugs— was transforming my interior into a chemical vat.

During much of my early illness I felt split into two selves, one the "sick" self I had to live *with,* the other the "normal" one I was trying to live *by.* I knew I had in some way to integrate them, but that was not easily done. A war was being waged between them until the healing could set in and the sick self could become the jumping-off point toward a new balance. I discovered ruefully that there is no "norm" to which the sick self struggles to "return." We live life forward, however perilously, although we retrace it backward, and after each travail we are lucky if we achieve a new equilibrium, never quite the one we left behind.

I began to see this as the essential nature of the healing process, by whatever agents it takes place—doctors, drugs, self, or all three together. Accordingly, toward the end of my chemotherapy, I wrote a reflective note in my journal workbook:

> *November 7, 1983* The chemotherapy enables the organism to find a new dynamic, which leads to a new equilibrium. . . . While cancer cells are dividing, others are now resisting them, in battle. Out of that resistance a new equilibrium shows itself which we call a "remission." . . . Illness is the failure of the dynamic to keep its shifting equilibrium in balance. Healing is the establishment of a new dynamic, a new equilibrium. Death is the collapse of both. . . . The entire process is and will always be a mystery, in a cosmos unheeding of us.

I might have added that death is the final equilibrium, the motionless one. Whatever was the prime mover in life, moves no more.

Since "equilibrium" has too much smell of stasis, my diary entry stressed the element of "dynamism." The organism needs both change and stability. When it experiences too sharp change, whether in itself or its environments, it gets thrown into disorder. It needs to reorient itself, establish a new pattern of order, before it experiences further change within that pattern.

Thus we move through the phases of the life journey, through crises and traumas to renewals. Severe illnesses, whether physical or mental, are of course the critical traumas. Even if they don't assume terminal form, they throw us into disorder, threatening our life patterns.

I add a later journal note from August 1987, headed "Re order and disorder in a metaphysic of healing":

> The thing we feel most in grave illness is the *disorder*. We lose our center of gravity. Our physiological body image gets distorted. Our whole being yearns toward restoring order. Hence the importance that our rituals of order assume, not only in sickness but in healing. I have in mind the rituals of sleep and waking, of work and play, of punctual medication, of the orderly patterns of the day which we are more likely to strive for in sickness—and in healing—than in unthinking health.

Emerson was right: "He has seen but half the Universe who never has been shown the house of pain." In the universe of the ill, I learned, there is a total narcissism of concentration on the negative symbols of self—sleep and sleeplessness, discomforts, bodily functions, ups and downs of mood, fears, pain, despair. The day and night are measured by needless, repetitive blood taking, doctors' visits, discontents with the attendants, and always a whole array of symptoms. You dread the coming of night with the narcotics that don't work and orderlies who don't answer your buzzer, with the groans of your fellow-sick as an accompaniment to the tumult of soul and body in yourself— along with the desolating loneliness of the long nights.

I was lucky, most of the time, to have a room of my own. But sometimes, as I listened to the angry voices in the next room, I wondered whether a sick man's quarrel with his attendants and doctors wasn't really his quarrel with God. Amid the contagions that spread in a hospital the worst is the mood of despondency. The sick pool their pain, grief, despair. The hospital has not yet managed to offer them a way to pool their hopes and affirmations.

One galling thing about the spells of chemotherapy was the immobility that went with my I.V. equipment. I couldn't move more than a few yards from it. I could do twelve paces back and forth in my room, and I traversed them for exercise, much as prisoners do in their cells.

When I went for tests I was wheeled through the crowded, draughty corridors in a chair, with my accompanying I.V. And there was the waiting—always the waiting—for doctors, for attendants, for tests, for their results. Often we were lined up in a row, the sick and old, in an array of wheelchairs. We were practicing the infinite patience of the ill, whose lot it is to wait in the antechambers of laboratories and doctors.

I thought myself into the minds of those who were sentenced to wheelchairs for life. It was not the worst imaginable fate, but it was a dark one. I thought of Franklin Roosevelt, who suffered and overcame it gloriously, and used his hard-earned command of self to command the nation. I thought also of Milton Erickson, who ministered a thousand therapies from his wheelchair. What counted was to retain your faculties of mind and imagination—yes, and to temper them in the crucible of waiting and pain.

It was conversations with my family and intimate friends that counted most for me. A dangerous illness can destroy family relationships if they are already crumbling, but it strengthens the valid ones. Illness has a way of sloughing off the inessential and causing us to focus on what comes first. Every

major illness is a combined tornado and earthquake, shaking
our values. You discover what was jerry-built in your life and
what can stand the storm.

I didn't, at bottom, believe I was dying. My journals were
crammed with ideas for articles and plans for new books that
belied my fears, real as they were. But most of my friends, and
perhaps my family, did think that death was near. Jenny has
told me since that this was true not only for the family but for
the "bystanders." "You looked as if you were dying," she related, "gray, shaky, thin, deflated. Add that to your look of
shock and your loss of your hair and you have the picture you
presented."

They were more scared for me than I was for myself. Somewhere within my inner terrain there was a spot I had chosen for
my fortress, and as long as I stood there I disbelieved in the
imminence of my death.

My initial round of chemotherapy came to an end. I was to
return to the hospital for a second course a few weeks later, and
after that I visited Dick Silver's office at periodic intervals for
doses of chemotherapy, while he monitored my white and red
blood counts for signs of improvement.

Like all busy New York specialists he had a number of examining rooms and he moved from one to another, disposing of
each of us with dispatch. Yet he was a demon researcher and
recordkeeper, always on top of his records (not all doctors are).
He was a heavy, square-set man, with a square face and a busy
manner. Despite his mask of gruffness he always had the necessary word of encouragement. He made me feel he was a devoted
ally in the ecology as well as oncology of my fight for life.

Doctors by and large disdain the role of teacher. Through
most of my chemotherapy I had only a hazy notion of how the
healing-poison potion was meant to work. Nor did the staff in

and out of the hospital try to enlighten me. Doubtless they were too busy. But perhaps also they feared that the mystery would be diminished, or maybe after the thousandth treatment they were just bored.

At one point Dick Silver decided to move me from a four- to a six-week schedule for my chemotherapy treatments. I expressed some anxiety, fearing that I would not be getting enough. He turned on me with more than his usual intensity. "Don't you understand?" he almost shouted: "It's poison I've been pouring into you! Be happy we can let up a bit. We give your body a better chance to do its own fighting." It was a little lecture I have not forgotten.

During the weeks and months of chemotherapy, I experienced a cluster of the expected "side effects"—nausea, dizziness, loss of appetite, loss of hair, numbing of my feet, desperate fatigue, depressive and manic moods. I didn't mind them too much, since most would be corrected, even the vanishing hair that hurt my pride. What I did mind was central: the sense of debilitation that affected the entire physical organism. Although briefed about many things, I was never told that, even with the best "recovery," I would carry aftereffects of the treatment with me to the end of my life. The lasting abrasiveness is the true case the "alternative" school can make against traditional surgery, radiation, chemotherapy.

Recently my son Adam wrote me a chastening comment on all of this, all the more persuasive because, as an oncology fellow, he had some experience by now with creating as well as administering chemotherapies:

I cannot argue that the chemotherapy experience was not a ravaging one. It may well live with you for the rest of your life. Yet while you praise the intellect of the scientists who created the LHRH analog injection, you do not reflect on how equally remarkable it is that, in less dramatic fashion, doctors have gradually developed a group of medications which in combination can cure many patients with the kind of lymphoma you had. It was an aggressive lymphoma and, after unpleasant and debilitating therapy, you emerged alive and apparently still full of a fair measure of pepper.

For myself, I am most amazed that it occurred as it did, and thankful to Jerry Barondess for his diagnosis and to Dick Silver for treating you so effectively. . . . I suppose that if I went through the experience myself I might feel less than wholeheartedly grateful to the medical-industrial complex and its attendant poisons and poisoners. If you do not sound explicitly grateful enough to the creators of the chemical coupound it is in retrospect understandable. . . . I think your answer would be that you were not simply "cured," but that you *and* the medicine licked the lymphoma, and that often it was as much you against the medicines as it was you against the disease.

It was a remarkably just comment from a young doctor steeped in the tradition of medical research and therapy, showing a penetrative balance that evoked my paternal pride. Yet he was also right about the tenor of my answer. It is exactly because our training and experience are different—his as an oncologist, mine as a patient with some longstanding chronic diseases—that our approaches (which have narrowed considerably) still diverge.

As I noted at the start of this book, this is a patient's-eye, not a doctor's-eye account. I owe much to the researchers who labored to discover and test the best pharmaceuticals, the best combination of chemicals. I wish however that those who came up with Adriamycin and Cytoxan for my advanced large-cell lymphoma might have hit upon a less bruising mixture, and I am certain that someday someone will.

I was scared enough about my life to take the harsher path of treatment because I also felt it was the more prudent one. The fact is, however, that we don't really know enough about failures, successes, and survival in the cancers, any more than we know about "success rates" in psychoanalysis. You make choices and live life forward and can't retrace them experimentally.

Even in the hard-wire figures on survivors, we don't know how much of the healing was due to the chemical, how much (as Adam noted) to the patient who was fighting not only the tumor but, to a degree, the doctors and even the chemotherapies addressed to the tumors. The ornery spirit, fighting the Adversary in every form, may be what releases the organic flow of energies.

If I had it to do over today I would do it the way I did. Yet if we had better figures on which to base our decisions, and more sophisticated ways of interpreting them, I might decide to take the alternative route. Someday we may have them. The cutting edge of the great advances in the years ahead is likely to be less with chemo-body than with mind-body and with hormone-body-mind.

5. Don't Take My Night Away

He calleth to me, Watchman, what of the night? Watchman, what of the night? The Watchman says: The morning cometh, and also the night: if ye will inquire, inquire ye: return, come.

— Isaiah 21:11,12

I have been one acquainted with the night.

— Robert Frost

We do not become enlightened by imagining figures of light but by making the darkness conscious.

— C. G. Jung

In the dark night of the soul it is always three o'clock in the morning.

— F. Scott Fitzgerald

I N THE BEGINNING . . . the earth was without form, and void, and darkness was upon the face of the deep." There are times in our lives when we re-experience the darkness and void of these opening lines of Genesis. And then, if we have the strength for it, we rekindle within ourselves the Spirit of God as it "hovered over the surface of the waters" and brought light into the cosmos.

Darkness and light are polar conditions of our lives, each stripped of meaning without the other. In the first years of my illness, 1981 and 1982, I had to live almost constantly with the darkness, but it was the struggle for light that enabled me to endure it.

Returning home in mid-March 1981 after my first round of chemotherapy, confined to our apartment except for visits to doctors and the hospital, I decided to set some short-term goals. I had lost thirty pounds and the effect had shaken me. I looked shrunken, crumpled. In an effort to mask the change, Jenny had my suits taken in and bought shirts with smaller collars. The result was scarcely an improvement, and I continued to lose weight in the early chemotherapy phase. It was an unhappy thought that while I ate, my tumor was eating me. Doggedly pursuing a high-protein nutritional program, Jenny stuffed me like a holiday capon, and in time I began to turn it around.

Another short-term goal, the effort to regain my elusive energy, was more disheartening. I had always prided myself on an unquenchable flow of it, a heritage doubtless from the sturdy stock of my ancestors, at once Jewish and Russian, who had endured hard ground for generations. But now, when I awoke, it took a display of will just to put on my shoes. By midmorning, when I most needed energy for writing, I would get drowsy over my books and papers. Gradually I learned how to pace myself and use my brief spells of energy. I also discovered that once I could start writing, the excitement of it generated more energy.

As a result I can't remember missing a deadline during my years of illness.

The heartbreak came from the havoc wrought in my teaching schedule. Early in January of 1981 I had done the first sessions of a cherished seminar in California, on Eros and the American Family, and had flown back to New York for a week's break. That was the week I got "the News" from Jerry Barondess. Phoning from my hospital bed, I had to arrange for staff associates to complete the quarter. The fact that they put their own urgencies aside to help me in mine was heartening for me. But another quarter was to start in April, and I was too involved with chemotherapy, and too weak anyway, to venture it.

This set my next critical goal for me. The first quarter of the new school year would start in mid-September. I was determined to be there. The interaction with my students and associates in the seminars was, I was convinced, critical for my recovery of self. If I gave up on it I would be giving up on life.

I wrestled with this specter, as I did with others, in the lonely watches of the night. I had been an untroubled sleeper, but now for several hours before I let myself fall asleep, my imagination became a battlefield. I had read just enough of the work of Carl and Stephanie Simonton, about their Houston cancer clinic, to be caught by their visualization idea. Their patients visualized the battle between the killer cells, who had taken possession of the field, and the benign cells whom chemotherapy was rallying to the defense of the organism.

Why not try it? Essentially it was cops-and-robbers stuff, a grim kind of play. I was playing at war, much as I had seen Michael and his younger brothers over the years, arranging their battlelines with their toy soldiers. I now made myself a four-star general in a map room, deploying the forces in both camps.

Yet amid the make-believe it was a real war I was playing at. I had a smoldering conviction of the reality of what I was doing as I ranged the battalions of cells against each other, then focused in turn upon each pair of combatants, and finally managed to make the forces of light smite the forces of darkness.

This diffusion of the boundaries between reality and imagination was playacting, yes, but it was willed playacting, a suspension of disbelief for high stakes. Playing the field marshal of these troops gave me the one thing I needed more than any other—the enacting of the drama of hope.

Hope was what it was about. In his "Ode to Dejection," Coleridge impaled it for me:

> Life without hope draws nectar in a sieve,
> And hope without an object cannot live.

The operative word here is "object." Coleridge was writing about a willed hope that aims at a longed-for event. These staged nocturnal battles were the road I chose to get back to my seminars by September.

I have no way of knowing what impact the nightly happenings had on the eventual outcome of my illness. Modern mind-body thinking is still in its infancy, and important research in what is barbarously called psycho-neuro-immunology started only in the last two decades. But in applying it to my own life I have learned to believe in it seriously enough to give it a chance.

One element of that seriousness is the way I tried to gather my resources, including the tags and pieces from a lifetime of reading. Every writer must remain a student of what I call the ghost faculty of his intellectual fathers, who support him in his time of greatest need. I recalled some of my own fathers in a later journal note:

We have banished the individual will by our mentally rigid and morally flabby determinism, whether of Marx, Freud, or behaviorism. I have tried to bring a few fathers back as allies in fighting my illness. They were the great commanders of the human will who gave it a central role in the ecology of the mind. (Friedrich) Nietzsche and his *will to strength* ("Whatever doesn't destroy me, strengthens me"). . . . (William) James, turning what the will commands into the daily practice of habit which in turn becomes ritual. . . . (Otto) Rank's *will of the patient* to rebuild his life, however damaged—even against the dogma of the analyst who calls it "resistance."

I decided to join these thinkers with a simple will therapy of my own, applying it where it was hardest, to a very physical disease. I had to fight the essentially passive role assigned to me, while all the artistry was left to the experts, the doctors and technicians. The very word "patient" (Latin root, *patior,* "to suffer") is a giveaway. Patients suffer things to be done to them, becoming thereby the *acted upon,* the diminished. We ignore the fact that patients have an intelligence, experience, and will of their own and can themselves be a resource in restoring the equilibrium we call health.

Rejecting this passive assignment, I spent the early months, in New York, seeking to restore a sense of the normal to my life. During the spring and summer of 1981, at Southampton, I worked and walked, and (weak as I was) surprised my friends by showing up at a succession of parties. They had mostly written me off, but there I was, a pretty scarred and shaken Lazarus, newly returned from the dead.

Perhaps to compensate for my relative immobility during the early years of my illness, my journals and notebooks began to

take flight. I voyaged in my mind, in part to convince myself
that these fluctuations in physical well-being were not damaging me as a writing and thinking reed. This may have been why
I started writing when I was scarcely out of the recovery room
after my surgeries, with the tubes still in me, planning articles
and books at my lowest moments.

The articles often remained unwritten, and some of the
books, alas, have languished. Yet the act of planning them was a
defiance of circumstance. "Every word we write," said Bernard
of Clairvaux, "is a blow struck at the Devil." The Devil for me
was the killer cells. Assailing the Adversary was the best therapy I could have hit upon. But even if I should fail, I also wrote
so that something of me would survive him.

I was still too frail to resume a lecture schedule, especially at
any distance. But when I was asked to talk at a synagogue
forum in New York I said yes, with the warning that I was
fighting a cancer and wouldn't be very spry. The crowd over-
filled the seats. Too weak to stand at the rostrum for any length
of time, I sat through my entire talk and the lively question
period, livelier than usual because it was the first year of the
Reagan presidency, which was my theme. After the last question I was whisked home, and I fell asleep with a feeling of
elation. This step led me to take on another talk, this time in
Detroit, which I saw as a preparation for my flight to California
in the fall.

If the days were an energy problem, it was at night that I had
to face the contingency of death, at night that I recalled events
from my crowded life which might never again be crowded. "In
the dark night of the soul," wrote Scott Fitzgerald, "it is always
three o'clock in the morning." It was during these three o'clock
nights that I retraced my talks with my doctors and mapped out
strategies to come. Nights can be formidable when you wonder
how many will be left.

Sometime in June, with a heavy sense of things moving too slowly, I decided that a change was imperative. Hearing that Dr. Mathilde Krim was doing some experimental work with Interferon, I reached her at Sloan-Kettering and found she was planning an Interferon program on lymphoma for the summer and was ready to take me on. I wanted to try it but felt shaky about switching from a protocol that might not be on the right track to one that had little or no track record. As I guessed, my doctors felt more testing was needed.

I yielded but made a counterproposal. My friend Morris Abram had told me that Dr. James Holland, at Mt. Sinai, had treated him very effectively years earlier for lymphoma-leukemia, helping to save him for a vigorous life. I was eager to call in a generalist for consultation, and asked for Holland. We compromised on a consultant from another hospital. Thus came the episode I have recounted in my opening chapter, when the specialist recommended a more aggressive attack on the tumor and gave me the honest but bleak six-month prognosis.

It was a low point in the erratic trajectory of my illness. But as I have noted, it galvanized me into a sharper, more urgent independence of action.

I remembered an episode in the early 1970s, in an Esalen workshop at Big Sur, when a colleague of mine grew eloquent about achieving a society purged of all its traumas and injustices. I recall turning to him and saying, with some passion, "Don't take my night away." For it is in the night of our being that we fulfill our nonrational needs, from honor to love to belief, and tangle with the sometimes tragic, sometimes absurd, fiber of our lives. If there is an affirmative side to the fact of pain and illness, it consists in our having to cope with them by calling on the perverse humanity of our sheer creatureliness, which is rarely elegant and almost always messy. *"Inter urinam et faeces nascimur,"* Freud used to remind his associates, borrowing the phrase from St. Augustine: Between urine and feces are we born.

I never quite made up my mind whether medicine as healing is a black art, full of paradoxes and antinomies, like chemotherapy, or one straining toward the light. Perhaps it is both. One thing I did learn from my experience: whatever the mix, you have to brew it yourself.

For me the six-month death warrant was a turning point as well. Even when accepting the compromise consultant, who fell short of my purpose, I had asserted an active role in the decision. If another crisis point came, on an issue I felt strongly about, I was determined to take charge.

I break my story for some words on what I learned—and was to learn—about the relation of doctors and patients. In our traditional perception of illness, the doctor has been central, the authority figure who notes the symptoms, maps out the test procedures, diagnoses what is wrong, decides on the treatment, superintends the healing. From time to time he may touch base with the patient but usually pro forma. The whole model is drenched with authority.

The patient suffers the illness, pain, disruption, and disorder of life. He suffers what is done to him, not as the subject of his own destiny but as the too passive object of the sometimes mistaken diagnosis, the endless testings, the medications and therapies, the minor and major "interventions," from catheters and biopsies to exploratory surgeries, radiation, bypasses, and transplants. He moves through technologies and ministrations alien to him, to a destiny he has had little role in shaping.

At some point I began to question this model. True, there was a time when my universe was in so great a disarray that I fervently sought the authority of a doctor who would bring order into it. Gradually I began to see that while I wanted attention paid to me, I would also have to pay attention to myself and bring my own order back into my universe.

It was more than an intellectual exercise for me: my life depended on it. I didn't mind being a "difficult" patient if that would help me define what role I could productively play in my course of healing.

In conversations with fellow patients, as we waited in the anterooms of doctors' offices, huddled together on wheelchairs outside the testing rooms, or walked and talked with each other in the hospital corridors, I was overwhelmed by their idolatry of authority. I saw their anxiety-ridden faces and watched the body language that conveyed the surrender of their sovereignty as persons. Among them were lawyers, teachers, executives, heads of families, community leaders. I wondered about their failure to assert their life experience and knowledge of themselves. My instinct was to distance myself from this mind-set.

For a time I clutched at the idea of a "doctor–patient partnership," with its accompanying "dialogue," which cropped up occasionally in more enlightened circles. It made considerable sense, since it recognized the need for pooling the resources of both agents in the illness-healing process. It was also a comforting concept. The term "partnership" carried with it a sense of fairness and equality, and "dialogue" has become a buzzword wherever pundits huddle to discuss "conflict resolution," whether in business, politics, marriage, or work.

I don't mean to downplay either the doctor–patient partnership or the existing dialogue between them. Both are to be cherished when they happen. But too often they are honored only in the breach by overworked, harassed professionals. Nor does the idea of partnership confront what occurs in the crunch, when the interests, viewpoints, temperaments, and values of doctor and patient clash. "When two ride one horse," wrote Thomas Hobbes on the question of sovereignty, "one must ride in front."

To the objection that illness and its healing don't involve a polity, I would have to enter a dissent. They do. Wherever you have a structure of authority, power, and decision making, you get clashing perspectives that need resolving. At that point you have a polity, whether a marriage, a hospital, a church, a university, a corporation, a government. In this sense there is in fact a government of illness and healing.

Which is why the idea of a true partnership, however seductive, remains difficult. The world of medicine has grown so complex that a patient without a good doctor is even more an amateur than a defendant who acts as his own lawyer. I strove for a genuine partnership and for a dialogue with my doctors, and they with me. But there was a critical difference between other partnerships and ours.

In the others, as in a marriage or other pair-bond, what counts is the relationship itself, good or bad, with stakes roughly equal. In a medical relationship the doctor has most of the knowledge as he fights for the patient's recovery, but the life-and-death stakes are the patient's alone. Hence the patient is the one who has to summon all the artillery of body, mind, and soul for the battle.

Let me change the metaphor. In the great drama of sickness, treatment, and healing, the doctor is on stage much of the time but the patient is center stage *all* the time, right up to the end, whether it is happy or unhappy.

I am not writing a Declaration of Patient Independence here, nor do I mean to sound me-heap-big-Injun. Few patients have more than an inkling, on their own, of the knowledge and experience needed for intelligent decisions. Most, like me, start as medical illiterates. The traditions of the profession call for the specialist or internist to deliver the verdict and recommend the decision, and for the patient to accept it.

The let-the-doctor-do-it model relieves the patient of incentive and responsibility. When we leave all the decisions to the doctor we surrender part of our fighting faith in our survival and healing. We may do it because we are awed by expertise, or because we think we don't know enough, or because we lack the courage to engage in a doctor–patient dialogue. But this model assumes a passivity on the patient's part which was alien to me. Within the larger frame of the doctor's medical authority I sought a measure of patient autonomy.

There can be no grandiose role here. It would be *hubris* for me (my parents would have called it *chutzpah*) to place myself above specialists who have devoted their lives to clinical practice and are in touch with current research, and to substitute my own judgments for theirs. No, the province of autonomy I sought was more modest, quite simply to inform myself—by every available means—to play whatever role came to me, because it was my life and my death.

Reading over my journals I am struck by how long it took me to assert this role. The torment of choice was pretty much what every patient with a dangerous illness endures. I had to learn how to resolve the often conflicting advice from my array of doctors and consultants, including my doctor son in Boston and my "behavioral medicine" son in Bolinas. At each crisis point they all became sources of "input" to balance against each other when there was a conflict between them. Nor did I mind if they didn't pull their punches. "If I want to hear someone's opinion," said Goethe, "it must be expressed positively; I have ambiguity enough in myself." I was in the realm of conflicting judgments and values. I needed the input to resolve my own ambivalence and end in decisive outcomes.

Once I had the assessments and recommendations of my consortium of doctors, I was the one who had to take charge. When a difficult choice had to be made, no one else could assume its burden. I had to carry it, not because of knowledge or experience but for the existential reason that my life was at stake.

My doctors recognized how much it meant to me to have the chance to disagree, as well as agree, with them. They knew also that a patient who becomes part of the decision process thereby becomes part of the healing process as well.

"Man," wrote Ernest Becker, "is a creature who denies his creatureliness." My spell of illness deepened my sense of man's creatureliness, but also of what man can stretch himself to endure and affirm. How can one peer into the heart of darkness and still remain spongy and tenderminded about it, substituting wish for reality?

There is a passage in *King Lear* where, encountering the Duke of Gloucester naked in the storm on the heath, Lear addresses him: "Thou art the thing itself! Unaccommodated man is no more but such a poor, bare, forked animal as thou art."

There were times during my illness—being wheeled through hospital corridors, shivering in a paper hospital sheath on a testing slab, waking from anesthesia in the recovery room— when the starkness of Lear's vision came home. All my "accommodations"—whatever I had gathered over the years to cover my creaturely nakedness—were stripped away. I was "unaccommodated man, the thing itself."

It was a chastening experience. Yet what also came through was the sense that I had a core selfhood—my mind and spirit, my life experience, my sense of my organism—to clothe me in the storm and cover my nakedness. For a patient who is sick and doubtless scared, out there in the storm, the very bareness of the heath is an irreducible starting point. Exactly because he has no "accommodation," he can shed pride and pretense, old conventions of thinking, new fashions.

So he turns to whatever source can help him: traditional medicine, "behavioral medicine," specialists, consultants, "second opinions," technicians, shamans. But since someone must take charge, who other than he, the sick one trying to heal, the one whom it's all about? As with Harry Truman on the Washington heath, the buck stops here, with the patient. For if he were no longer here, there would be no buck.

The summer was a hard one. My doctors split on the consultant's program for adding radiation to chemotherapy. I cast the deciding vote against it. I followed what my organism was telling me, that it had taken the roughness of chemotherapy and didn't want to add that of radiation. It wanted a chance to show what it could do. Besides, while I had an imagery for the battle of the cells, I had none for radiation.

What my organism told me must have been on target, because by early September our joint efforts began to show results. The white blood cells, too low all along, started to shoot up, a sign that my system was recovering from the damage the chemotherapy had done to my bone marrow while killing the cancer cells. My treatment visits to Dick Silver were producing some good signs. True, my spleen was still distended, but my energy was returning.

Then I got a different message from Silver. The new problem, he said, was that after a while the tumor develops immunity to Adriamycin, so some other treatment had to be found. On that score, time was running out.

Yet, however weak, I was determined to fly to the Coast. It was a payoff, as it were, for my efforts at a sustained will therapy. My voice was fragile and husky, but a microphone could make up for it. I was gaunt and feared I would scare my class. But I never doubted that the expense of effort would set the energy in me flowing again. My doctors, understandably skeptical, had little choice but to humor the intensity of my decision.

As the summer waned my journal blossomed with ideas for

my first seminar. In mid-September I flew to Los Angeles. I worked as usual on the plane, and my journal noted that I "got my own bags on arrival" and spent several days in L.A. before I flew on to San Diego.

A work-plan footnote: I was flying to a series of seven-hour teaching weekends, divided between Friday evening and Saturday morning, with a group of perhaps 100 doctoral students in the behavioral sciences. The seminar was mine to plan and conduct but I shared the lively student discussions with several faculty associates.

When I walked into my class (that quarter the seminar was on "Change, Renewal, and Innovation"), I was stunned to find in the rotunda, rising row on row from the rostrum, more than 150 students, a few standing in the aisles. Everyone had turned out for my homecoming, whether out of passion for learning, or curiosity, or to make sure they wouldn't miss what might be my valedictory message.

I felt so moved that I was rattled and overtalked, "I threw too many questions about change at them," my journal notes. But in the classes that followed during the quarter I got my bearings again. When some of the students threw back really barbed questions at me I knew they had lowered all the protective guards and meant business.

My journal (October 1) sketched out some overambitious future writing on reassessments of the presidents of our century, starting with Franklin Roosevelt. At the end I jotted down a note: "I must stay alive to do these books. I must. . . ."

Looking back now, writing not with a doctor's but a patient's eye-view of the difficult dynamic of recovery, I can discern some of the experiences I traversed in getting to this determination to "stay alive." I trust that they may to some degree parallel the stages that others are passing through, whatever their illness.

I start with the initial shock and pain. Although they were both realities, the pain has since almost receded in my mind. Some memory of the experienced traumas, however, still remain. The body in pain is always a reminder of mortality, even when the threat of death is absent. The long night watches in a hospital, with pain as a constant companion, were themselves tolerable, except for the question of how many nights like them would follow.

Our dream may be of a world in which pain for the ills of the body will be abolished, yet its association with the human condition would still be there. "Pain has an element of blank" was how Emily Dickinson put it. We all know the intense point where one gets dissociated from it, almost as if it were an abstraction. But unless we know pain in our own experience we cannot feel with those who know pain at the hands of others. Our creatureliness must persist if we are to retain our fellow-feeling.

The experience of shock is more vividly present in memory. "My first feeling," a friend who had a massive heart attack told me, "was that my body had let me down, I lost control of it. Despite my friends I felt terribly alone." I noted earlier that I too had the sense of having lost my center of gravity. Things were topsy-turvy in a universe that made no sense.

Both the pain and shock, although inherently disorienting, took on an added dimension from fear. I have had shocks (of death in the family), and I have had pain more intolerable than the tumor in my gut. But they were finite. In this case they loomed larger because of the fear of what they portended, a fear that compounded the pain and shock. It is the lion in the path whom every sufferer must confront.

"This can't be happening to me," we say. But it is. "Things can't get any worse," we say. But they do. The downward descent becomes a vicious spiral. In my early cancer days, the tumor was eating my food as well as me. Every time I found I had lost weight I dreaded the next weighing, and my dread, along with the killer cells, became a self-fulfilling prophecy.

If I had to recall some episode of fear which is symbolic of all the others, I couldn't think of anything grand and impressive. Mine was slight, with an everyday banality. I had come home after my first round of chemotherapy, and Adam was taking a break from his Yale Medical School studies and keeping an eye on me. I felt pretty shaky, with a sense of mistrusting my whole neural system, along with the chemical vat within me. Something might happen, I didn't know what.

One evening Jenny took a breather from her watchfulness to see a play. I had Adam and a friend of his as dinner companions, but they too had a movie date. Just as they were leaving I got a sudden gust of panic and asked them to call off the film and stay with me until Jenny returned. They did.

I ask myself still—as I did then—what I was so fearful of. Obviously death that might come not as some grand climax but in the midst of life's routines. "Men fear death," wrote Francis Bacon, "as children fear to go in the dark." Here I was, at eighty, guiltily asking my grown son to stay home, as a child at bedtime begs his parents not to leave him in the dark.

I was afraid of the "dark." More nakedly and simply, I was afraid to die. Or rather, I was afraid of some unknown happening in that scarred system of mine which might strike without my having someone there to help me in my need. Illness brings dependence, as childhood does. But while a child grows out of it, the dangerously ill don't know when or whether their dependence will end, short of death.

It is easy to admonish someone else to banish fear, and there are times when it works, as when a political shaman called

Franklin Roosevelt told his countrymen that "the only thing we have to fear is fear itself." In the case of the human organism, the patient may try to play the shaman himself, to exile his fears.

The trouble was that mine were grounded in a reality that couldn't be conjured away, the stubborn *facticity* of both my tumors. There is also the fact that fears accelerate the pace at which the reality worsens, and that too is a reality of its own. So I was caught between the two realities, the tumor and the fear. I see it now as a stage of Purgatory, not after but before my descent to my Hell, an antechamber of Hell.

The tangled question of stress, introduced into the modern discourse on health by Hans Selye, is now accepted as one of the sources of the onset of cancers and heart attacks, and an energizer of the process. Of course, the stress involved in fighting stress can and does beget a stress of its own. I had to deal with that paradox in my own healing. I regret now that I didn't make the effort to learn some "relaxation" techniques like yoga or meditation. So I met stress as the enemy and improvised my own ways of struggling with him, only to find (as others have) that the enemy was myself.

Thus my calendar of pain, shock, fear, and stress, singly and together. I now feel, looking back, that there was no way to end this war early. In the bleak early years of my illness, when we all felt I was losing my battle with the tumor, I had first to reach the bottom of the mineshaft within myself.

Jenny later provided some details of the despairing mood of that period. She enlisted a close family friend, and together they ventured into the chaos of my study, sorting files and folders, getting pyramids of books off the floor to make room for a hospital bed she planned to buy, and organizing the place for me to come home to die. She knew I would want it to happen among familiar and loved surroundings, not in an alien hospital room.

I knew only dimly of these preparations. But how could it have surprised me, even if Jenny had been more explicit? The consulting lymphoma specialist expected me to die within months, and two lawyers came solemnly to my hospital room with a copy of my new will to sign, and Jenny and I chose my literary executors. My daughter Joanna Townsend flew in from London for what she hoped would not prove a farewell visit. My daughter Constance Russell, in San Diego, held long phone colloquies with me on life and death as we examined our past relationship. My close friends on both coasts expressed their affection in what I described in my journals as an "elegiac" mood.

I wanted no elegies. "Sing no sad songs for me." I wasn't dead yet. True, I was scraping the bottom. Yet even in the darkest days I never stopped feeling I could somehow start the arc of health moving upward again. I felt it in a tropism of conviction that seemed to come from wherever the springs of the life force rise and flow.

No, it wasn't a "placebo effect," nor was it a "Lazarus effect." I was not innocently benefiting from some experimental elixir whose true nature was hidden from me, nor was I returning from the realm of the dead. Call it a *touching bottom effect*. When I touched bottom, I had to burrow inside, to turn my being around toward healing.

6. "You Are Twice-Blessed: You Have Two Cancers"

When Sorrows come, they come not single spies
But in battalions.

— *Hamlet,* act 4, line 78

Give me health, and a day, and I shall make the pomp of emperors ridiculous.

— Ralph Waldo Emerson

Wovon man nicht sprechen kann, daruber muss man schweigen.
(What one cannot speak of—about that one must remain silent.)

— Ludwig Wittgenstein

You just have to take a white-knuckled grip on life.

— Rick DeMarinis

ANY NARRATIVE OF an extended illness must somehow reckon with the task of reconciling subjective feelings with objective states. I sensed this at the point in my illness when my friends began to comment on how well I looked. "I look better than I feel," I had in candor to answer, "and I feel better than I am."

One might call it the presentation-of-self effect. We present ourselves best to others in how we look, and next best to ourselves in how we feel, but the crunch must be sought in how we *are* actually in our functioning.

The discrepancy may lie in an internal communication lag. Each of us is like a backward country: it takes a while for messages from the primitive interior to reach the capital. My subjective mood often remained dark, a carryover of a struggle, even when in fact my white blood cells were on the rise. At other times my mood was sunny, even when the signals of threat and danger lurking in my organism—in the belly of the beast, as it were—had not yet reached my perception.

There is a tradition in German literature of the *Döppelgänger,* the double that exists somewhere in the world outside us, the polar opposite (or Jungian *shadow*) of the self we recognize. This was true of me for a spell, when I seemed to lead a double life, in the fall of 1981. My California seminars went well. So did the series of lectures I give every fall at the New School for Social Research, in New York. My writing and teaching were beginning to cohere again—and I thought I was too.

My journal at the time expressed something of this:

> My remission continues, with five-week intervals between medication. Sleep, weight, and energy good. I think I have passed the hump and should have another 2–5 years, perhaps as many as 7, even without total remission.

It was a way of staking out a claim on the future.

Yet an entry two months later reflects a more astringent mood, as if a dour message were trying to get to me.

> I write this at midnight, just as I reach my 79th. It has been a terrible year, the worst of my life. . . . Aside from the cancer and surgeries there have been weeks of setbacks: my shingles, the operation for the hernia, the nosebleed that became a hemorrhage, the general malaise. A few days ago Jerry said there is no objective change in my illness—that it has to be subjective. I said if that is all then I can handle it . . . I feel this will be my great testing year, and if I make it I can go on for a time. . . . I face my 80th in not such good shape, but a damned sight better than if I hadn't begun to mend three months ago. More wryly I say, Happy birthday, Max.

Ten days later, on December 29, 1981, there is a note of guarded hope:

> Good developments. . . . Both doctors are reasonably optimistic. Radiation will be only one option, back-up drugs possible. . . . I'd like to get to 85 if not longer. . . . Have an offer for a visiting chair in American Studies at Notre Dame, starting in the fall. Donald Costello is flying in next week to discuss it.

So I did the winter quarter at San Diego and took up the offer of the chair at Notre Dame, to start the following fall. I looked forward to a year's adventure there and planned to return to my California teaching when it ended.

I was still troubled by doubts about the future, however, and in an effort at least to secure the past I had a sudden urge, toward mid-February 1982, to write an autobiography. By mid-

March I had written 150 pages! "Very excited by it," my journal
records. "A torrent of memories." I was determined not to be
overtaken by death without having left some account of my life.

But I didn't reckon with the actualities of the present, which
were competing with the memories of the past. I shall return to
the theme of the autobiography and the ultimate healing role it
played. But a brief journal entry from March 18, 1982, in-
troduces another, more sinister player:

> Not so good on the illness. A month or so ago Jerry
> got worried about lung spots. They are real. Dr.
> James Smith did a bronchoscopy but failed to get the
> tissue they needed for study. Jerry rightly decided
> against surgery. We are all—including Dick Silver—
> up a tree about finding another chemo. I am seeing
> Dr. James Holland tomorrow as outside consultant.

Behind those staccato jottings there was a tangled story, il-
lustrating how a new turn in an illness may elude the skills of
very good doctors and throw the case into a frustrating blind
alley.

It all began with an X-ray at the start of September 1981,
showing a "cluster" on one lung, which seems to have awak-
ened little concern. This was probably because we shared what I
now see as a lymphoma mind-set, and a fleeting lung spot
seemed irrelevant.

Not until February 1982, five months later, did worries
emerge. Dick Silver, I noted in my journal, "hears things in my
lungs," and so we all went back to the early September X-ray—
and took more—to see what might have caused Silver's suspi-
cions.

This time a lung specialist was called in, Dr. James P. Smith,
and his reading of the X-rays confirmed that something was
indeed happening in the lungs. But what? Had the lymphoma

spread? If so, it would require a new chemotherapy, and none suggested itself. Worse, it might be a tumor of the lung itself.

That thought blanked out everything else. When Jenny and I left Dr. Smith's office, our mood was wintry as the weather. My willed cheerfulness and the illusory sense of well-being that had sustained me threatened to go up in smoke.

I had to face the new dark possibilities. So I asked again for a consultant and insisted that this time it simply had to be Dr. James Holland, whom I had not fought for hard enough the previous June.

Thus began my second descent into the maelstrom of uncertainties. It differed from the first descent, however, in a critical respect—my attitude. I had lost my innocence. I was determined this time to be clear-eyed and unillusioned. I would pay due attention to doctors, tests, and all the paraphernalia of medicine, and especially to the views of my new consultant. My doctors knew more than I did. But in a crisis of conflicting judgments I would never forget that the final, critical decisions were mine to make.

Jenny and I found James Holland in his setting as a working hospital doctor, in a cluttered huddle of examining rooms on the fourth floor of a shabby converted apartment building. It served as an annex to Mt. Sinai Hospital and at that time housed the unit on neoplastic diseases which Holland headed. It was a far cry from the state-of-the-art presentation I had expected.

I sat for a time in a seedy waiting room filled with a Whitmanesque array of whites, blacks, and Hispanics of every class and condition. There were Harlem matrons, aging Orthodox Jews wearing yarmulkes, a trade union official I had known years ago, a well-dressed South American couple who had evidently flown in for a consultation with the world-renowned doctor. When my name was called I passed through a crowded treatment room filled with people getting their chemotherapy injections, who were chattering in a spirited way with the attending oncological nurses. It was a scene I liked: no silent people with tight faces, no sanitized assembly-line atmosphere, but very human beings in a workshop of healing. (I have to add, as I write, that the annex has been replaced by a new hospital building, with a neat, orderly array of examining rooms and laboratories. It is splendid in its modernity, but I feel a nostalgia for the original.)

In one of the examining rooms the man I had been seeking since the start of my illness rose to greet me. How describe him? If I had expected some Carlylean, haloed hero-as-physician, this was not he. He was slight physically, in his fifties, totally alert, eyes twinkling behind his glasses. I felt that he came at me as if he sought to burrow into the self behind my seeming.

I could have wished for a Picasso to draw him, with all the lines and angles intersecting to express the rich contradictions of the man. The face was at once open, sympathetic, engaged, dispassionate, quizzical, absorbed, amused. Always (as I was to discover) it carried authority, always it conveyed an image of total immersion. At that moment, I felt, I was the only person who counted, because for that moment I represented the particular of the larger issue Holland cared about most. For me he had—and has retained—the charisma that goes with earned authority. No Dante about to be inducted into the circles of the Inferno welcomed his Virgil as fervently as I welcomed this guide through the Hell, Purgatory, and Paradise of my illness and health.

He took my history swiftly and skillfully, pouncing on details no one else had singled out. Then he put me through a scrutiny more intense than I had ever experienced. Nothing was left uncanvassed. There was no cranny, crevice, orifice of my now blotched and misshapen body that he didn't probe, firing a battery of questions as he worked. I welcomed it, since a lifetime of clinical experience with every variety of cancer went into this history taking and organism probing. I recognized the generalist in the specialist and felt that every question had a line of direction. He was treating me as a whole person.

When I had dressed and felt that my body was back in my possession, he gave Jenny and me a first overview of his findings. It was a rough approximation in a quite literal sense. Seeing me as a very sick man, he pulled no punches.

His initial hypothesis, like that of my other three doctors, was that the lymphoma had spread to the lungs. He drew the logical conclusion—that I must shift to another and more effective chemotherapy. What was new was his confidence that there was one available for me, since he had used it to good effect with a number of patients.

Sobering as his view was, I didn't act on it immediately. I was getting to be a warier, tougher bird, if also a more riddled and beset one. It felt good to have Holland, with his experience and authority, as a resource on what was emerging as my doctor "team." But I was beginning to fancy myself as a novice producer of my own drama. I wanted as close to a consensus as I could get from my doctors, and I was not yet ready to hand over control. I had another round of talks with them, but couldn't find enough agreement to act on.

The thing that puzzled me was that we all had a sense of crisis, including myself, yet I was not feeling like a patient in crisis. I was feeling remarkably well for a battered old specimen! And all the clinical indices that Dick Silver pursued so sedulously, including the white blood count, continued to show an upward arc.

I returned to Jim Holland in April 1983, roughly a month after our initial encounter. He made it clear that the X-rays he had now seen—and my own witness about how I felt—had changed his perspective. He now saw the center of gravity of the case shifting radically. The shift shed doubt upon the assumption which Holland had earlier shared with my doctors and me, that the clusters on the lungs were the product of a spreading lymphoma. He still felt that a new drug might prove necessary, although we couldn't make any decision without knowing the source of the tumor. He wanted to see all the scans and get a new lung scan.

The critical thing now was to extract some tissue from the lung. During the month between my visits to Jim Holland we had all been wrestling with that one—how to get a snippet from the lung without cutting me open. James Smith finally did a bronchoscopy at New York Hospital on one lung. It was a delicate procedure, not without pain, but it didn't produce the fragment we all wanted. We talked of a second try, but there was little reason to believe it would succeed where the first had failed.

By now we had moved into May. During the winter I had said yes to Donald Costello and the offer of a chair at Notre Dame. When the lung complication arose I grieved about having to forgo my seminars for the spring quarter in California. Now I had to confront the prospect of reneging on the Notre Dame agreement, since I couldn't give Costello the assurance that I would be well enough at the end of the summer to start my teaching.

Costello eased things for me by saying that the agreement still stood, whenever I could make it, if not for the coming university year then the one after. It was the first breakthrough of hope in what had been a bad season. I readily pounced upon my new short-term objective, to be well enough to start my Notre Dame teaching by the end of August.

As I saw it we had two tasks. One was to decide the sort of procedure we needed—major or minor—to get the tissue for analysis. Until we did that we wouldn't know the source of the cancer that was causing the "clusters" on the lungs, if indeed it was a cancer. Meanwhile we had to decide what kind of chemotherapy I should be getting for my existing (and continuing) lymphoma until we made that finding. It came close to being a classic double-bind situation.

The only way to break through the bind, I felt, was to continue the conservative course until we knew more. Dick Silver had not yet reached the allotted end of the Adriamycin protocol. He urged completing that course, reasoning that, aside from the lung clusters, my improved performance justified it. Jerry Barondess agreed, as did I. It was a case of choosing to continue treating the symptoms we understood until we could discover more about those that eluded us.

I was still unhappy about the tissue-for-analysis issue. Jerry Barondess had been reluctant about surgery from the start, and recalling my spleen fiasco I blessed him for it. Yet now there was no alternative. We had to resort to surgery—minimal, I hoped. Dick Silver opted for a "thoracic biopsy," and Jim Holland suggested a "Chamberlain" procedure via the upper chest. Jerry Barondess acceded and chose a thoracic surgeon.

So, with anything but a light heart, I entered New York Hospital again, only to find, in talking with the surgeon, that he felt a Chamberlain wouldn't get at the lower lung. What he planned was a full-scale surgical entry, sawing a rib to gain access.

I was dismayed. Was this the "minimal" procedure my doctors and I had agreed on? It was not. Yet there I was again in the hospital, being prepared for the knife the next morning with no warning, and with no time to call my council of war together.

I didn't blame the surgeon, whom I had never seen before and who was undoubtedly giving me his best judgment. But I was enraged and I expressed it in a presurgery journal entry: "I feel as if I had been—with the best of intentions—sandbagged." I thought we had developed a plan for collective decision making, and suddenly it was swept away.

It was a bad night for me, and the morning would be coming soon, and everything had been arranged, and there seemed to be no going back. I felt trapped. I could say with the narrator in T. S. Eliot's poem, "This is not what I meant at all. This is not it at all!"

Was I being unreasonable? I had been through too much surgery of this sort to wish for more. My prejudice against major exploratory surgery was based, I suspect, on my image of a whole body being wheeled into the operating room and a mangled body emerging from it. The image kept careening through my mind during much of that troubled night. Surely, I reflected, there are better ways to run a railroad if you must have an exploratory track.

My journal entry two days later was in a shaky handwriting:

Praise Whoever presides over a universe of Chance! My "biopsy" went well although more severe than I had thought. . . . Dr. Okinaka made a long incision below the nipple, to the right near the armpit, took out some rib, got at the tissue he wanted. I was away over four hours but the procedure took 1½–2 hours. Today (a little over 24 hours later) I am a battered old hulk with a resilience that surprises everyone. The

> frozen sections showed "probably no lymphoma but
> some malignancy." The doctors guess it may be "low-
> grade." The hope is that some chemotherapy may
> reach both cancers. So after 4 or 5 months of contest-
> ing and struggling I am in a new phase. If I don't
> survive the next year it won't be for lack of battling.

Now that we had the tissue, the problem was to discover what it said to us, beyond a "low-grade malignancy." What was it exactly? What was its source? What was its relation to the lungs? These queries ushered in another month of testings, probings, explorations.

The prevailing guess was that the prostate was the offending source. But when my urologist did another biopsy—he had done one some years before—the results were again negative, to everyone's disappointment, since a prostate tumor is slow in growth and can be treated.

By this time it was August, and with Jerry Barondess away on vacation the understanding was that Jim Holland would keep surveillance over me. Along with his knowledge of cancers, I had found his general diagnostic judgments bold and tenacious. He showed these qualities again, refusing to give up on his prostate hypothesis despite the negative report on the biopsy results. He wanted "more information" before acting, and he meant to act. He asked for all the X-rays, scans, and pathology studies from diverse sources, including the tissue studies after the lung surgery, to pass through the eyes and judgment of his pathologist at Mt. Sinai.

His parting admonition, as I left for my Notre Dame teaching, was to remain confident that, one way or another, we would get out of the cul-de-sac of paralyzing uncertainty. I recalled the old Roman phrase from my freshman Latin studies: *Sursum corda*—"lift up your hearts!"

To arrive finally at Notre Dame, after six months of travail over the lymphoma and the lungs, was some sort of triumph, if only of a dogged stubbornness. It was even more a tribute to my total medical "team," which, despite persistent uncertainties and delays, was functioning with some harmony.

My work plan for the year was to commute every two weeks between New York and South Bend, which would keep me in touch with my doctors. My classes, on the changing American civilization of the past quarter-century, marked the first time in eight years, since Brandeis, that I taught undergraduates. My faculty associates were generous and able. The campus was an idyll. The youth and ardor of the students renewed my own.

Jenny came with me. In formally assuming the new chair I delivered an inaugural lecture for faculty and alumni on American civilization studies. The next day, in a whipping cold breeze, we watched the opening Notre Dame football game of the season with Father Theodore Hesburgh ("Father Ted"), the university president. It felt like a brave new world for someone so recently mangled in the hospital.

In my journal entry I find a summary of some of the themes in the inaugural lecture:

> *September 18, 1982*   I dealt with what we are all *un-done* by, what civilizations live and die of, my criteria for a healthy society, the self-woundings of a young civilization rather than the terminal sickness of an old one. To the question of whether we are a dying civilization, my answer from *Porgy and Bess:* "It ain't necessarily so."

Obviously the undercurrents of my conscious and unconscious mind had affected my metaphors about the state of the civilization. Or perhaps the two simply flowed together.

Philosophically I was a possibilist on both the personal and the collective fronts. To the determinists, whether Marxist, Freudian, or behaviorist, who hemmed in the sphere of our action, my answer was the willed assertion of the life force against the Adversary.

I start and end with the conviction of man's imperfection and the frailty of the tenement he inhabits. But (with William James) I recall the splendid taunt of Shakespeare's *Henry IV* to Crillon, "Hang yourself, brave Crillon! We fought at Arques, and you were not there!" Whatever happened, I had fought at Arques and, however bruised, had learned from the experience.

In a break between my Notre Dame classes, the last week of September, I went to see Jim Holland again. While we sat talking, after he had examined me, his phone rang. He listened for a while, said "Good," and then, "He'll not be displeased to hear it."

It was the head of surgical pathology, Dr. M. Kaneko, calling with "good news." He had studied the lung slides taken at New York Hospital and ruled out both the colon and the thyroid as the source, along with the lung itself. This was the news which had evoked the "He'll not be displeased to hear it," and I breathed relief as Jim relayed it to me.

"It's curious to congratulate someone for having a prostate cancer," he said, "but I do." I understood his meaning. It was a better source for the lung clusters than any other because, however troublesome, it was manageable.

He turned back to the phone, and from the conversation I gathered that the pathologist wanted three "blank" (unstained) slides from New York Hospital in order to stain them, and wondered whether I might have difficulty getting them. Holland assured him I wouldn't. "He's eighty," I heard him say, "but he has the tenacity of a bull."

I felt flattered and told him so. His smile was mischievous. "You are twice-blessed," he said, "you have two cancers."

So with my two cancers I was to count my blessings! But clearly I couldn't do it simply by willing it. I see this episode now, however troubling, as another stage in my renewed struggle for recovery by stages. Call it the working-through stage. The fact that I had already experienced the agony of "touching bottom" helped me now to work through the curse of helplessness to a feeling of control, work through near despair to a sense of possibility and even confidence.

It was a long stage to traverse, with many little backsliding defeats as well as victories. Much of the time I simply coped with the urgencies of the day, without feeling that I was embarked on a high strategy. I came to measure time by the varied faces it presented to me, like a river which swelled and diminished, depending on the ups and downs of illness and healing. It was Time in Henri Bergson's sense of *durée,* not divided into a neat democracy of equal units but reflecting in its *duration* the varying intensities of my organism's journey.

During my clouded period, as I have noted, I started an autobiography. It was just about the time my doctors became anxious about the "cluster" or "cloud" on my lungs, in mid-February 1982, and failed in their efforts to get at the source. My mood and motives were ambivalent. In part it was an act of cosmic balancing: if my life-as-experienced was drawing to a murky ending, I could at least contrive another to take its place, my life-as-remembered. I wanted to rescue a brand from the burning, however charred. It was a stagy gesture against oblivion.

So I dug out my earliest journals and read through bundles of old letters, and mined my recollections. It was a bittersweet experience, at once painful and exhilarating. In writing about my Yale undergraduate years, for example, I got down to some long forgotten memories of how my grand Yale classmates, the sons of the rich and mighty who ruled the world, shut me out of their glittering universe as a cocky little New Haven Jew. The exhilaration came from rediscovering memories, as in an archaeological dig, peeling away the layers of rock and dust to reveal the hidden residues of long repressed feelings.

So I worked on it for six or seven months, from February to the early fall, the narrative flowing swiftly, much as a kaleidoscope of lived events is fabled to flash through the mind at a moment when life threatens to end. I had some 500 handwritten pages and had reached 1945—age forty-two, in the midst of my stint as a war correspondent.

I left it hanging there, where it is still hanging, not (I trust) for too long. What happened was that the confusion about the lungs began to clear, and I started my Notre Dame teaching, making the present again viable and the future less uncertain. Mining the past was no longer the prime urgency.

Yet I now see, more clearly than I did at the time, how integral it was to the working-through stage of my healing. What had started as a gesture against death, and of resistance to oblivion, took on an unanticipated role in my self-healing, and thus in the affirmation of life.

I pause again for a backward look on my illness to ask what the path was that led out of the wilderness to a clearing of some sort. The working-through effect I have mentioned, how did it *work* for me?

An analogy may be useful. In tracing the evolution of life, cosmologists speak of a *food chain* linking the common fate of living things: when it broke at a critical point, its effects were felt all down the line. So the principle of connectedness applies to the total human organism.

A possible metaphor is that of a *sickness chain* which operates with some sort of domino effect, as a dysfunction in one system exerts an adverse impact on others closely connected.

But if a sickness chain why not also a *healing chain,* in which the return to functioning in one system exerts a positive effect on the others?

The domino image, with its implied principle of momentum, comes to mind. Granted, this isn't some impersonal principle of physics we are dealing with but a living organism. Yet in that organism the test should be not only in what happens on the downward slope, which is apparent enough, but on the upward slope, which researchers are only now starting in earnest to probe.

Just as I felt a downward domino effect in the turmoil of my clouded phase, so I felt a positive domino effect in the elation of the upward arc of healing. When I stopped losing weight during my first cancer and started to gain without food forcing, I had the pleasure of curbing my mounting appetite by a somewhat rational regimen. My new-found energy took me outdoors in walks, wood gathering, and tasks around our grounds. This helped my digestion and made me sleep better, without nightmares. The energy I got from walking and sleeping in turn enabled me to work more productively. My concentration improved, words came to me more readily, my imagery grew more confident. The memory losses that accompany illness and aging seemed minimized. My web of relations became closer and stronger.

Every new advance built on the sequence of all previous ones. I seemed to be on a euphoric binge. My work became more playful; my play allowed more scope for the mysterious processes of work. I had always tried to break down fences between work and play. I now found it easier to keep the fences from forming. The reality for me was something very like a reversal effect. After the shock and anguish, the stress and pain, the anxiety and fear, the bottoming out and the slow ascent, I began to have the feeling of putting it all together.

It is hard to fix on the exact occasion when the will to live asserted itself with a confidence that brooked no self-doubts. It was not a one-time thing that sprang full blown. In my most troubled illness years, after a note on some long-range project, I would jot down a phrase in my journal: "I *must* live."

I can't recall when the "must" became "I *can* live," turning resolve into possibility. It was the wager phase, a time when I hung on Dick Silver's battlefield despatches as he reported the results of the blood tests. I would sit in the examining room, writing, but actually waiting tensely, watching his face as he entered the room, to detect what the smile or frown augured. I was like the Victorian reader who bought each issue of the magazine to see whether Charles Dickens or Anthony Trollope would kill off a character or let him live. It was life-or-death by installments, only in this case it was my own life.

The turning point came at one visit to Silver when the nurturing cell count moved upward. So did my heart. I noted it in my journal that day, and added, "I didn't take the bus home. I walked." It was my way of celebrating. The good news gave me the right to walk despite my weakness, but the jubilant walk in turn did wonders for my mind and doubtless for my cell count.

I couldn't will my mood out of the blue because I couldn't get away with fooling myself. But I could use some nurturing event to build a mood without feeling foolish. That was how I used all my good news.

Not all of my healing course had calm waters to sail on. There were hopes, but also dashed hopes. There were signals of increasing energy and also setbacks. Dick Silver, with all his encouragements, was careful not to raise my hopes, lest the fall be steep. Yet the auguries continued favorable, and the time came when I reached a new phase in my conjugation of the verb "live." After moving from "I must" to "I can" I took the final step. "I *will* live" I told myself, and while the element of sheer resolve was still present in "will," it was fused with an element of confidence I had not dared earlier.

How and when did this feeling come? The episode was so minor that it appears an anticlimax rather than epiphany. It centered on the opposite bank of the East River, which runs past our apartment as it also runs past the hospital a half-mile farther downtown. I used to stand at the window of my hospital room, looking across the river at the cars, buses, people. I watched them with envy. I once had their vigor. I would not have it, I thought, for long. Back at home, still struggling with my first cancer, I looked out every day over the same river at scenes on the other bank, still with envy tinged with sadness.

Then one day much later, when my lung complications were starting to resolve, just about the time I decided to put away my memoir and return to my ongoing daily work, I noticed something. As I looked out at the opposite bank, at the river and the tugs, it came to me that I no longer was sad about them, nor did I envy the people I saw. Instead I felt elated. I was part of them and they of me, part of the same enterprise of life which flowed out of me into an indefinite future, as the river flowed.

7. "Don't Let Them Do an Abelard on You"

We sail within a vast sphere, ever drifting in uncertainty, driven from end to end. . . . Nothing stays for us. This is our natural condition and yet most contrary to our inclinations, we burn with desire to find solid ground and an ultimate sure foundation whereon to build a tower reaching to the Infinite. But our whole groundwork cracks and the earth opens to abysses.

— Blaise Pascal, *Pensées*

The Gods of the Earth and Sea
Swept through Nature to find this Tree;
But their search was all in vain;
There grows one in the Human Brain.

— William Blake, "The Tree of Life"

To the destructive element give yourself and it will bear you up.

— Joseph Conrad

WHILE I WAS HOSPITALIZED for my lung surgery my son Adam, then an intern at Boston City Hospital, had visited me. He was our "scientist" son, in a family that was mostly involved with "soft" pursuits like literature, psychology, journalism, and the human disciplines. At Andover he had read the poets and edited the school paper, but once at Amherst he discovered the enchantments of biology and research. He had reached out toward chemistry and physics and the rest and gone into medicine—to the delight of his mother, who saw in him a reprise of her own surgeon father.

We talked for three or four hours. Our takeoff point was Werner Heisenberg's "uncertainty principle" and the entire complex of quantum physics which proved unsettling even to so bold a mind as Einstein's. *"Der liebe Gott,"* he said, *"würfelt nicht mit dem Universum":* Our dear God doesn't play dice with the universe.

That (I told Adam) was exactly what "der liebe Gott" has been doing with the contingencies that brooded over the universe of the ill. Yet I thought I knew what Einstein was driving at. While he was not religious in any traditional sense, he had spent his life discovering the true laws of Nature. For him, Nature's God was both Lawgiver and Lawkeeper. He couldn't tolerate uncertainty. There had to be underlying order, even if man, at any given moment, might not be able to discern it.

Jim Holland knew this about his cancer patients. Much of his healing art lay in seeking to dispel uncertainty. That explained the wryness behind his "twice-blessed" remark. I had tolerated one cancer and could tolerate two. It was a relief to know that the lymphoma had not spread to the lungs, since it meant that the first cancer was more or less contained. Although it was a blow to learn that I had a second cancer, I could take that, too, if it proved treatable.

When Holland's pathologist, Dr. Kaneko, stained the three

slides, there was no doubt left that the source of the carcinoma discovered in the lungs was the prostate. A number of times during the course of my illness I had occasion to note the difference between routinely competent therapy and resourceful therapy. From start to end, the manner in which Jim Holland pursued the prostate as quarry was the resourceful brand.

The question now was the age-old one of how to treat it. "What can I do about it?" I asked Holland. On earlier occasions, when hard decisions had loomed for me, I recalled his admonition: "Above all, don't panic." While I didn't panic this time I can't deny I was a bit scared.

I should have been a fool not to be. Prostate problems are frequent for men in their seventies, and usually they yield to surgery. But I knew that prostate cancers are different. Even when they are "indolent" they can kill. What emerged from the literature and from masculine lore was the unlovely choice between dying and losing your masculinity.

There was no great emergency, Holland told me. He had known patients who rushed into action and were later sorry. He laid out the possible options. The nub of them all was to diminish and finally all but eliminate testosterone, the male hormone, which was (alas) the source of the tumor's growth. This could be done radically by castration, or less drastically by estrogen, the female hormone.

Both methods were reasonably effective, said Holland, although the cancer often returns. Estrogen had the disadvantage of a feminizing consequence. Surgery would be psychologically brutal. Given what he had gleaned from my life history and our conversations, he could see strong arguments against both.

"Decidedly," I agreed, a bit grimly. "Is there a third treatment?"

A year or two ago, he said, there wouldn't have been, but I was lucky in my timing. There might be a better way now than the two he had presented. It was an analog of a newly discovered hormone called LHRH. Two American scientists, Andrew Schally and Roger Guillemin, had received a Nobel Prize for discovering it. A constant administration of LHRH was meant to reduce the secretion of a pituitary hormone necessary for the production of testosterone. A West German pharmaceutical company had made the new hormone available to Dr. George Tolas, in Montreal, who used it for an experimental test group with good results, as reported in the *New England Journal of Medicine.*

Could I get in on it, I asked? If I decided on reflection to take that route, Holland answered, he didn't see why not. He would call Tolas. But I might have to establish residence in Canada.

We canvassed each of the choices. I had no enthusiasm for growing female breasts and even less for having my genitals excised. In fact, I was dismayed by the thought of either. Whatever their physiological effect, the psychological one would play havoc with my self-image and with the willed energy that kept me embattled against the cancers.

We both knew I would be having discussions with my team of doctors. Holland's own status was still that of a consultant. He would write me a formal letter laying out the alternatives, with his recommendations.

As he left the examining room he half-turned and aimed a parting word of advice over his shoulder. "Don't let them do an Abelard on you," he said.

His words touched my literary nerve more sharply than he could have guessed. I had read the story of Heloise and Abelard in adolescence and had returned to it in my teaching years. One of the prime histories of the tribulations of desire and love, it told of the young twelfth-century scholastic theologian, Pierre Abelard, of Brittany, who had jousted with the church authorities and been condemned for heresy, but attracted a swarm of students from all over Europe to his teaching at Paris. Among them was Heloise, niece of the canon of Notre Dame. They fell in love, Heloise had a child, and they were secretly married. But her kinsmen came in the night and exacted their revenge on Abelard (as one account has it) "by inflicting on him a shameful mutilation." In the end Abelard became a monk, Heloise an abbess, and their conjoined spiritual and carnal love became one of the grand myths of Western romanticism.

The fact that LHRH was still experimental caused me little concern. It was almost a plus in my calculations. From the time my first cancer had surfaced I had sought to bypass the traditional therapies and try the innovative ones. Now at a critical point in my struggle for health, I had a chance to act out my convictions.

Jim Holland sent me his formal letter as consultant:

I am pleased to tell you that the immunoperoxidase stains arrayed on your pulmonary biopsy by Dr. M. Kaneko, head of surgical pathology at Mt. Sinai, have disclosed positive . . . evidence that the tumor cells contain prostatic acid phosphatase. Thus the diagnosis of metastatic prostatic carcinoma is unambiguous.

I relished the technical language as a wrapping for the punchline to come:

We have previously discussed the treatment options, which are expectant observation, castration, stilbesterol administration, and the possibility of an LHRH analog. We are just beginning studies with this last agent, and the results in a few patients studied in Canada and Europe are extremely promising. My general inclination would be to advise you to do nothing as long as you can, and then, with scrupulous avoidance of the fate of Abelard, consideration of LHRH or diethyl-stilbesterol.

It was a splendid letter, its boldness executed with care, its final imperative reviving the drama of danger in the Abelard story. It put the burden of decision where it belonged—on me—but in such a manner as to give me ammunition to try the experimental way.

It was ammunition I needed. My doctors followed the medical canon of reluctance to embark on a still not fully tested treatment when traditional tested ones were available. I didn't blame them. But as a patient I had my own canon and my own priorities.

After touching base with them I talked the alternatives over with my doctor son Adam, in Cambridge. I was delighted that he had read the report in the *New England Journal* and found it, for all its tentativeness, a weighty one. He was young and inexperienced, but he was developing a *gravitas* of judgment. I was moved by the dance of the generations which had a father asking for the counseling of his son.

I had all but made my decision, yet things kept intervening. My Notre Dame classes were demanding, the commuting schedule difficult, and in addition I had agreed to take part in a conference at the university on the ethics of the media, chaired by a new young professor friend, Robert Schmuhl.

Then, on one of my visits early in November, Jerry Barondess prodded me sharply. After three months the new X-rays of my lungs showed that the lesions were worse. "Let's get cracking," Jerry said.

It was a good reminder and as an incorrigible delayer I badly needed the prodding. Jim Holland was abroad, and I had been dragging my heels intolerably. When I saw him on his return a few days later and told him I was ready to start, he must have sensed a residual quaver in my intent as we talked about possible side effects. Thus far in the experimental use of the analog, he said, they were minor.

"I think you should do it," he added. "It can't do you any harm. It can only do you good."

This was what I needed to take the plunge. But when I talked with Dr. Tolas there proved to be difficulties. I had hoped to make my initial Montreal trips during the intervals between teaching, take my work along, and do my writing between treatment sessions. Tolas agreed to admit me to the experimental protocol. But while I had assumed this could be managed with the immigration authorities, their verdict was that as a noncitizen I would have to establish residence in Montreal for a number of months.

This dismayed me. I had counted on a Montreal stay during the winter recess only, but three or six months would doom my resolve to finish my Notre Dame year. Besides, my heartbreak over missing the rest of my commitments might cancel out whatever good the Montreal treatments could do.

Again I played in luck. During my delay of several months Jim Holland and others were negotiating with the Food and Drug Administration and the pharmaceutical company (in New Jersey) for permission to start an American experimental protocol with LHRH. In my last conversation with Tolas he suggested I might find it easier to wait for the release of the drug to the American group. Holland gave the same advice. It might take several months, he said, but the negotiations with Washington and New Jersey were promising. I could then be one of his first patients in the American tests.

I had muddled through to triumph. It was exhilarating to know I could both continue with my teaching *and* start my new therapy. My next week at Notre Dame was the last of the semester, before the holiday break. A journal note, written at Notre Dame, reflected my new mood:

December 8, 1982   I managed last night to do the notes in time for my last class of the semester (Is the Civilization in Decay?), ended lecture and discussion

by ten, bade my students Godspeed—only to see Don
Costello & the American Studies family come march-
ing in with cake, wine & candles, and Don gave a
graceful 80th birthday speech, &—wholly surprised
and overcome—I responded much too lamely, & the
students all gathered around & gave me birthday
cards, & then we adjourned to the Faculty Club until
II. It was a delight and I count my blessings. It has
been a glorious semester and done much to save my
life.

Happily, the winter recess that came with my chair was a
long one, and I was spared the arduous Midwest weather. So I
set off for California again, where I wrote in the sun during the
day, sat in front of a log fire at night, and gave some lectures on
weekends. The friends with whom I stayed were indulgent and
stress was minimal. Even without treatment my second cancer
seemed muted, as if grateful for the cosseting it got.

I returned in early March to my classes, happy in the knowledge that Don Costello and the American studies faculty had
confidence enough in my health and teaching to extend my
appointment for a second year. This bolstered my own confidence that I could weather the new cancer.

In March, also, came my induction into the hormone therapy. It came in the form of a vial of Buserelin, the pharmaceutical which the Hoechst laboratories furnished to the American
protocol. I was one of a little group of Jim Holland's patients
waiting for it at Mt. Sinai. His chief oncological nurse introduced Jenny and me into its mysteries, with Jenny watching the
injection in case I ever needed help.

I didn't. It was good to discover I wouldn't be tied to a hospital but could do my own daily injection into my thighs, alter-

nating them, with a needle whose length made it seem more formidable than it was. I came to enjoy it, gruesome as that sounds, not because the hormone was addictive (it wasn't) but because my visualizing faculties were brought into play. I re-enacted my psychodrama scenes of my first cancer, but this time the images were less gory and more beneficent. With each injection my imaging mind followed the course of the Buserelin, to the pituitary gland and then down to the testosterone.

Curious about what was meant to save me from the dread traditional therapies, I did some research. The men responsible for the hormone were Andrew Schally and Roger Guillemin, both working on a theory that linked the hypothalamus, in the brain, with the pituitary gland in the endocrine system. They were bitter research rivals, bent on outracing each other to a Nobel Prize. Working in separate laboratories, both began crushing masses of animal hypothalami to extract the precious hormonal stuff. I proved to be the beneficiary, among others, of the mountains of sheep brains and pig brains that were thus sacrificed. Reluctantly, the two scientists shared the Nobel. In my universe, the concrete result was the synthetic derivative of the hormone they had isolated, called the LHRH analog for short.

Over the months, as the symptoms diminished, my lungs cleared. I had been spitting up blood earlier, but now I stopped that. My prostate, on manual examination, grew less swollen.

During this period I acquired an accomplice. Enter Dr. Vincent Hollander, an endocrinologist in the Holland contingent (the names are only accidentally similar) who was to take charge of me in the LHRH protocol. He reminded me of Dickens's Mr. Pickwick, at once benign, tolerant, and shrewd. Since that March day in 1983 he has examined me in regular sessions, keeping track of the hormone effects and watching for any signs of new or returning cancers, or any symptoms that would affect my basic health.

He is observant, caring, unflappable, with judgment as his strong suit. He knows more about me than most doctors would care to know. Yet he retains an amused tolerance of my succession of symptoms (which have generally led nowhere) and an undimmed belief that somehow his warder's task will weight the balance of life against death.

So the early months of my injections of Buserelin sped by, as we waited for signs of the effects. They came sooner and better than we could have hoped. A journal entry from July 7, 1983, conveys my elation at the tell-tale lung X-rays:

> Vincent Hollander showed me the lung X-rays before and after a 2-month-plus spell. There was a dramatic change. Jim Holland saw them two days ago, with a 3-month range, and was also impressed. The blood-spitting from the lungs, which lasted about 6 weeks, is long ago gone. The prostate is diminished. "It is still largish," said Hollander, "but if I were checking it for the first time I wouldn't say we needed a biopsy." Even Russell Lavengood (my urologist), who has watched over the prostate for a decade or more, even before the cancers, called it "normal." Jerry Barondess agreed that over the space of 3 months the change was marked. . . . Lo, the hormonal drug has worked for me! They gave it 6 months, after which they would abandon it if it failed, and it took only two or three to succeed! Whatever else happens—and I am not yet out of the shadows (the lymphoma may reassert itself)—the prostate-lung carcinoma connection

is on the way to being resolved. And without castration!

Two friends and contemporaries of mine, who had prostate cancers at about the same time I did, were less lucky and less happy. Both underwent castration. One was a few years older than I, the other a few years younger. I shall call them X and Y. My journal for July 7 continues:

> I visited X the other day. He was bitter. "Max," he said, "they cut out my balls." I also met Y on the street. His whole look and bearing—the way he walked, the way he held himself—had changed. He said, "I am not Norman Cousins. I am not brilliant. I can't take over my own treatment. The doctors said, 'You have a prostate cancer, and the thing to do is castration.' What was I to say? They ought to know."

Y was a talented, accomplished man, of considerable distinction in his field. Yet he was still caught in the myth of the absolute authority of the medical specialist. It didn't require "brilliance" to dispel that myth, only the use of his own intelligence. The doctor's vocation requires inquiry, scrutiny, verification, judgment. The layman needs to check on the experience of friends, get second opinions, have some notion of what he is getting into. There are people who spend more energy and intelligence finding an apartment or buying a car than on weighing life-and-death decisions.

What is the nature of the healing dynamic that operates for us all? We are part of an ancient tradition that goes back before the rise of modern medicine, to folk medicine, the shaman, naturepathy, and the "perennial philosophy." We are also the beneficiaries of a movement of very modern energies. I am thinking of laboratory research in the life sciences on the brain and its "messenger" connections with other systems. I am also thinking of exploratory work in the human sciences which seem only distantly related to medicine, yet enrich our understanding of ourselves as healing organisms.

I know of few idea movements where so many have been drawn in to help so many, and whose common currency has come out of the incandescence of fellow feeling. Yet despite the broad base and the benevolence, something disciplined will prove enduring in this new view, call it psychosomatic, holistic, integral, or behavioral medicine, or call it simply the mind–body connection. That "something" will have to be validated in the end, both by experimental evidence and clinical experience. In that sense we are in the only province which counts in the advancement of healing, the province of disciplined rigor exercised in the service of the innovating imagination.

Do we sense something like a *healing hypothesis* emerging all around us, which we can draw on? If so, it centers on the mind–body connection, which I regard as the holiest of all Holy Alliances in the domain of human health.

As with all alliances, there are quarrels over which is the prime partner. The "somaticists" say the body, the soma: unless it offers favoring circumstances and means, the mind alone will be helpless. The "mentalists" see the mind as in the driver's seat: unless it takes charge the body will go the way of all flesh. It is a futile argument in a marriage of interacting and equal partners.

What turns most people on, making them converts to the new view, is less the wonder at how the soma works (we have been into that for centuries) but how the mind, psyche, emotions, and life style work to bring on disease or to effect healing.

The question of "cause" is likely to remain obscure. In my

own case, I had some notion of a sharp shock in my emotional life that could have triggered the lymphoma. But I had other signals—of working, traveling, stress, and food habits, and of environmental factors—that could equally have done it. Alas, I can't relive my life to test the causative hypothesis.

While I added an affirmative program of my own to the intervention of chemotherapy, I am now certain that I could not have managed to survive without the chemotherapy. But could chemotherapy have managed it without the healing chain of the therapeutic resources of mind? I would have to say *no,* even though I can't prove it.

The chief actors in the healing drama taking place within me were the brain and immune system, and the cells within both whose receptors were the central messenger system. Every supportive message, however shaped, that passed through the brain cells on the way to the immune system, strengthened its capacity to fight the hostile events that trigger illness. Every responsive message in the intricate circuitry of these "pathways" in turn lightened my spirits. The process worked for me in the healing of my lymphoma and again of my prostate. It is still working its effects.

One thing I learned from my experience was not to stretch the healing hypothesis too far. The mind–body connection is not an abstract formula but a set of possibilities, to be pursued in the context of the shaping episode or critical therapeutic event from which everything else must start. That event carries with it whatever is available in state-of-the-art interventions and technologies. Prudently chosen and wisely used, they become the start of the healing dynamic.

For my lymphoma I used the available chemotherapy; for my prostate cancer I chose the Buserelin hormone injection. When the chemotherapy showed results, however bruising its side effects, it joined with my subjective self-therapies to give me a grand start toward healing. When the hormone analog showed its splendid results—in this case with only euphoric side effects—the same mind–body fusion carried me far toward healing.

This doesn't mean that the only healing is self-healing, as some enthusiasts claim. I couldn't have reversed my first cancer without chemotherapy as a start, nor the second without the hormone as a continuing palliative.

The proposition needs to be put differently: not that all healing is self-healing but that there can be no healing *without* self-healing. It is the age-old distinction between the necessary and the adequate. As part of the knowledge revolution we are learning more about the brain, the immune system, and the endocrine and neural systems than we have yet been able to turn into viable healing concepts.

In Elizabethan times William Harvey expressed his sense of wonder in an apostrophe to the heart and its workings (see Chapter 9), with language more lyrical than any physician today would dare address to the brain or the immune system. Had the Greeks developed their science far enough to see the importance of both systems, they would have made gods of both. We make a god of neither. Instead we currently hyphenate the critical research areas into something we call psychoneuro-immunology, abbreviated PNI, thus fobbing off our sacral impulse. In time the hyphenating and abbreviating will doubtless find other forms, but they may not bring us much closer to resolving the ancient riddle of healing.

No small part of that riddle is the role of the intangible we call spirit and soul. I was on a euphoric binge, transported into a state of being where I was tapping levels of consciousness long dormant while I struggled with the grubby creatureliness of survival itself.

Actually, what I was experiencing may have been a form of autohypnosis. I knew of the masterly work of Milton Erickson in helping people to achieve "altered states" through medical hypnotherapy. Yet I didn't take it seriously until my frolic with my own succession of altered states. Every chronically ill person, I am convinced, has this experience of slipping forward into a changed state of being and then back into the accustomed one, without being able to name what has happened. For whatever obscure reason I resisted hypnosis at the time, I was wrong. I would have fared better with guidance like that of Erickson. Fortunately I managed on my own to slip back and forth, in a Captain's Table routine, between the altered and habitual selves to which I was bigamously married.

It was heady stuff, part of the aspect of healing that doesn't get much recognition.

One of the happier byproducts of the revolution in health consciousness has been to bring the antique concept of soul back into current use. In earlier years, while teaching seminars on selfhood and its components, I would move from *soma* to *brain* to *mind* to *psyche,* elaborating on what differentiated and connected them. During my healing phase, as I stood at the blackboard for another go at the same question, I found myself, after *psyche,* adding *spirit* and *soul.* I had not planned it, yet somehow, having written the added words, I knew that after the experience I have described I could do no other. In a different way each stage moves through what physiology, neurology, logic, and psychology study, to a realm that transcends them but remains an important component of the total person.

During the ailing/healing years, I learned that the healing reality is not suspended in midair. Along with the network of neural receptors and messengers it has as base a spiritual reality which is grounded in survival but reaches to belief of some sort. The nature of that belief varies with cultures and theologies: the fact of it is common to all, just as the shamanic tradition, which joins spirituality and belief with healing, is found in some form in almost every culture.

The historian of religions, Mircea Eliade, noted that the shaman had himself often suffered a deep illness and in combatting it had been drawn to healing others. A similar insight may be found in Carl Jung's archetype of the "wounded healer." The common theme is the creative force evoked by illness that has been noted in the lives of great thinkers, artists, political and religious leaders.

One thinks of Charles Darwin, with his intolerable headaches, charting the evolution of man; of Sigmund Freud, with his cancer of the palate, invoking the life force to counter the death principle; of Milton Erickson, paralyzed, using hypnosis to animate the frozen psyches of patients; of Stephen Hawking, totally immobilized, spinning hypotheses of unification theory for the cosmos; and on a political level, of Franklin Roosevelt, also strapped in a wheelchair, teaching a fearful nation to recover its energies and walk.

It was an image never far from my thoughts. Every patient, as Albert Schweitzer saw, carries a doctor, as healer, within himself. Everything connected with illness is a wounding experience. It is an inspiriting thing to think of both patient and "doctor within the patient" as part of the healing process, and to see both as using the healing to recover from their wounds.

8. A Medical Miracle– and a Medical Museum

A ticket to Heaven must include tickets to Limbo, Purgatory, and Hell.

— Henry David Thoreau

Anxiety receives us like a Grand Hotel.

— W. H. Auden

We all understand more than we know.

— Blaise Pascal, *Pensées*

What doesn't destroy me strengthens me.

— Friedrich Nietzsche

I TURN TO AN INTERLUDE in my story which was far from edifying, but which most patients will recognize as going with the territory of illness. I was coming to know the inner world of the sick. Much as I tried to detach myself from my body and direct my attention outward—to my writing, classes, notebooks—I was constantly pulled back to the body, my body. It was almost as if it were jealous of its rivals for my attention.

I was more battered by the cancers than I knew and suffered from a plethora of marginal symptoms. At one point my journal listed them: "edema, skin rash, weakness of walking, lack of energy, stiffness of body—and therefore concentration on symptoms." A few days later there was another note in a similar vein:

> William James kept talking of "healthy-mindedness," in his *Varieties of Religious Experience*. All very well for him! I wonder whether he would do it if he felt encased in all the curses Dad and Mother used to wish annually on Pharaoh. . . . This flurry of symptoms threatens to drive healthy-mindedness out of my mind.

My possession by symptoms should have been scarcely surprising. I was paying the price for two and a half years of tests: X-rays, scans, medications, procedures, biopsies, bronchoscopies, major surgery, chemotherapy. Scarcely a week had passed without one or another invasion of my organism.

At one point I got a nasty edema in both legs. Jim Holland feared a phlebitis, which could have dispatched me for good, and was all for bundling me straight off to the hospital to be bandaged and watched. Happily, no room was available, so I went home to bed. The alarm had been raised however and I had to cancel my spring seminar. Yet later, when I flew to Europe with Jenny, my feet became so swollen that I contemplated an immediate return to the safe haven of home and doctors. I stuck it out, although what walking I undertook in London and Paris was a painful hobble. In time medication and a more normal routine of functioning stabilized me. Yet the episode was a reminder of how vulnerable I remained.

One of the carryovers from the first cancer and the chemotherapy was the dependence I developed on prednisone, a counter-drug to Adriamycin. It was an antidepressant, and it saw me through some of my dreariest days. In fact, at times Jenny described me as subject to "compulsive euphoria." When I stopped the chemotherapy I cajoled my doctors into letting me continue on prednisone. I reveled in it for almost two years until Jim Holland, checking my regimen, urged me to get off it. Its dangers as a steroid, in side effects on the heart and elsewhere, were too substantial to gamble with.

I dropped it, only to experience a sharp loss of energy and bouts of depression. I felt guilty, not only because it was a dangerous dependence but also because it might interfere with the clarity of the hormone effect. So I cut the dose in half as a temporary bridge, and then again in half as the final bridge, and I gradually learned to live without a drug crutch.

There was no letup however in watchfulness. While we were monitoring the prostate and its promising behavior, the ghost of the first cancer haunted us. Was it in remission? Would it suddenly return? The consensus pronounced it a thing of the past but no one could be certain.

There were also intimations of possible new cancers. At one point a mystery pain led to a series of scans, but a hypothesis of a cancer of the pelvis proved fruitless. At another point the threatening sign was "hot spots" on a bone scan (raising the specter of a bone cancer), but Jim Holland was skeptical, suggesting that the scan had been misread, which proved true.

I had to learn the hard way, via a series of tension-producing alarms, that the universe of the ill (especially with cancers) requires a constant watchfulness, married to a skepticism just as constant.

Meanwhile the cancer of the prostate which had kicked up such a fuss was submissively healing. Each time Vincent Hollander went through the ritual of checking on the offending organ, he rendered his verdict with a sense of wonder: if he didn't know its history, the prostate would seem normal for my age. And each time this was dulcet music to me.

In December 1984, twenty-one months after the start of my protocol, Drs. Holland and Hollander presented me at Grand Rounds at Mt. Sinai Hospital to several hundred doctors, residents, and staff. "I am proud of your vigorous recovery," Holland had written me earlier. "Let me know whether you can make it and if not I can look around for someone else, although perfection has no imitation."

I needed little persuading. His epistolary style was a bit on the flamboyant side, but in presenting my case at grand rounds, his language was professionally technical and economical. When he finished, Dr. Holland introduced me. I spoke of my warm relations with both doctors, but expressed my conviction that the patient can help best by following what he knows best, his own organism, and claiming his final vote in the decision-making process. I thought I detected some fleeting quizzical glances among the audience.

There has to be an element of triumph in a recovery from a dangerous illness, and I didn't mind savoring it. Given what the sick go through to reach the Paradise of recovery, there is little enough vainglory in it. Thoreau as usual put it best: "A ticket to Heaven must include tickets to Limbo, Purgatory, and Hell."

When the two years of the hormone protocol were up, in March 1985, Vincent Hollander and Jim Holland recommended that the treatment continue. The testing of the experimental group was still too recent to serve as a base for certainty. Why give up the hormone when it was working? Why not go on, instead of risking a return of the tumor? Beneath Hollander's almost casual tone there was a note of tension.

"Go on how long?" I asked. "To the end of my life?"

"Yes, to the end of your life."

So I shall continue to give myself the daily injection that has already eased and lengthened my life.

I sometimes wonder about the element of contingency in the whole episode. What if my tumor had come earlier, before the German and Canadian testing results became public? What if my doctors knew nothing of it and didn't exert themselves to find out? And the affordability issue: what if I were like so many who are excluded from experimental programs because they lack the money and have no doctor who will put them on his list? Our fate lies, I fear, in what the conditions of our lives have made of us.

Reading an interview with Andrew Schally, the man who isolated the hormone, I made an unsettling discovery. "It's not a cure," he said. "It has to be constantly renewed or the tumor will return." So that was why my doctors had sentenced me to the injection for life! If I had any illusion of total recovery someday, that ended it. A conversation with Vincent Hollander confirmed my new insight. So I live with periodic sonograms of the prostate, hanging on the hope that the process set in motion by mounds of sacrificed sheep and pig brains will continue to be effective.

The final test of all research is what happens in the patient's universe. Mine continued in good shape. Schally said that among the outcomes of LHRH there is a possible antidepressive effect, and a release of energy and appetite. God help me, I must testify to the truth of this. I was energetic, I ate ravenously, and I bored all my friends with my unending euphoria.

There were more flashpoints in the continuing saga of my illness, which came (in 1984 and 1985) in tracking down a sequence of elusive symptoms. They raised questions about the return of one or the other of the old cancers or the emergence of some new one.

At a point when we had chased one problem through a number of failed hypotheses, I remarked testily to Jim Holland that I had just about lost patience with this temperamental organism of mine. Holland was examining my lymph glands at the moment. My journal of December 5, 1985, notes his amused response: "You are a medical miracle, and it is my privilege to keep you alive and healthy. But—you are also a medical museum."

How could I deny either of the appellatives? At Grand Rounds, Holland had presented me—on the record of my healing—as a miracle of sorts. But on the parallel record of symptoms I knew he had hit upon a home truth: I had also become (and I winced at the knowledge) the curator of my own medical museum.

9. "Thank God, It's Only a Heart Attack!"

The heart ... is the beginning of life; the sun of the microcosm ... by whose virtue and pulse the blood is moved, perfected, made apt to nourish, and is preserved from corruption and coagulation; it is the household divinity which, discharging its function, nourishes, cherishes, quickens the whole body, and is indeed the foundation of life, the source of all action. ... Every affection of the mind that is attended with either pain or pleasure, hope or fear, is the cause of an agitation whose influence extends to the heart.

— William Harvey, *Motion of the Heart*

The heart has its reasons which reason knows not of.

— Blaise Pascal, *Pensées*

In the desert
I saw a creature naked, bestial
Who, squatting upon the ground,
Held its heart in his hands
And ate of it.
I said, "Is it good, friend?"
"It is bitter—bitter," he answered;
"But I like it
Because it is bitter
And because it is my heart."

— Stephen Crane

DON'T TAUNT THE GODS. They have better ammunition than you, are quicker on the draw, and besides they are lords of the territory and control all the communication routes.

I learned this to my sorrow. I had weathered the prostate cancer and was holding it in check. My lymphoma had not returned. I had completed the fall 1983 semester of my second year at Notre Dame. During the long break between semesters, on one of my frequent visits to my longtime friend Hugh Hefner—always memorable for their carefree serenity—I worked in the sun at Beverly Hills on some faculty lectures I was to give at Notre Dame in the spring. I relished the prospect of the years ahead, in a universe where the ills of body were endurable, and the joys of mind and spirit seemed favoring winds for this rickety, barnacled vessel of mine.

Again, I reckoned without my old royal adversary—contingency. Toward the end of 1983 I woke in the night with a sore throat, a high temperature, retching stomach, and alternating chills and sweating. In the early morning I reached Jim Holland in New York, who guessed rightly that I had a pneumonia and commanded me to board the next plane out of Los Angeles, promising to see me at Mt. Sinai Hospital. Jenny met me, and by evening a resident attached to Holland's unit was taking my history.

The next couple of weeks were nasty. In addition to my pneumonia bacillus I became host to another, but unwanted, gift of the hospital environment. To counteract this I was given a second antibiotic. Alas, it happened to be exactly the one which had felled me in another hospital years earlier, and gave me a severe case of hepatitis. My body broke out in rashes, and even as I traded quips with Holland and Hollander, who like Rosencrantz and Guildenstern were in spirited daily attendance, I railed against hospitals and fate. At the low point of the combined pneumonia and hepatitis, I was convinced that malady would follow on malady in a vicious sequence, and I would never get out of the hospital alive.

In retrospect I now see the episode in some perspective. Cancer patients are threatened not only by the cancer itself but also by the infections which may hit them because of the punishing effect of the cancer on their immune systems. This explains why Jim Holland took my pneumonia seriously and moved so swiftly to get me under the surveillance of his neoplastic unit. The immune system message carried by the pneumonia bacillus was clear to him, and he was taking no chances. But unfortunately the same immune system vulnerability which brought me to the hospital laid me open to still another bacillus.

In time I recovered and was back at Notre Dame until May, adding a series of faculty lectures on the history of the presidency to my undergraduate ones. After another batch of late spring seminars in California I returned to our country house in Southampton to savor the summer there as Jenny and I have done for over forty years. This time Jenny took advantage of the radiant fact of my recovery to let me fend for myself, and she made a trip to London and Wales with our young grandson, Joshua Lerner.

Even alone, life seemed good again, and order had been restored. It was early July 1984, and the weather was heavenly, its sunny days and cool nights joining to complete the harmony of my life.

I spent my days writing, I watered the gardens and brought in wood, and sometimes on evenings which invited a fire I ate my dinner before the fireplace and declaimed on the joys of life to whoever would listen.

It was a summer idyll. I felt so good that the long chatty letter I sent off to Jenny in London, detailing my uneventful pursuits and my late-night musings between dream and waking, ended with a florid passage about the delights of my "still frail vessel" as it "careened on a hypnagogic sea."

One night, early in July, I dined late, sat by the fire reading and writing, and went to bed around midnight. Bed turned into a battlefield of violent, sweaty, and turbulent wakefulness. I had to get up repeatedly, bathed in sweat, to towel myself down. Even worse, I had a sense of increasing constriction in my chest.

Determined not to panic I rationalized my inordinate sweating as due to my hormone injections, and my chest constriction as indigestion. It was the blunder of explaining the unfamiliar in terms of the familiar, of following past stereotypes instead of responding to a new situation. If I was having a heart attack—the thought flashed through my mind—where was the expected stab of pain in the arm? Had I been less ignorant I should have recognized the symptoms as preliminary events to the main bout. The truth perhaps is that deep within I did know, but cognitively I didn't know I knew.

So far my luck with my heart had been extraordinary. It was a doughty heart, and I thought of it as an invincible ally. Hadn't it seen me through a long, demanding life and then through five years of insolent illness? It had served as well as Don Quixote's nag, Rosinante, in carrying me through my life's wars. Should I now surmise that it would itself fall victim to the wars?

I didn't give that fleeting thought enough credence to call for help. It was now after 2 A.M. I was alone in our old country house. I could call and waken friends, doctors, summon an ambulance. But during my illness I had zealously followed up many symptoms without result, and I didn't want to raise a fool's or weakling's alarm. So I half-dressed and went downstairs in a bathrobe to read, compose myself, and wait it out, whatever it was.

As I was sitting doltishly, like an animal of the plain waiting for the hunter, the telltale message came soon enough—a sudden pain in the upper left arm, not a sharp stab but noticeable enough. Along with the chest constriction and sweating, it was, I knew immediately, the thing itself.

I was finally spurred to action and phoned Mary Johnson, our family internist at Southampton for forty summers. Trying to avoid panic I spoke casually—"I think I may be having a heart attack"—and gave her the symptoms. I was to dress, she said, and an ambulance would be there in fifteen minutes.

"I don't want an ambulance," I said, "It's too big and noisy and it scares everyone, including me. I'm perfectly able to drive myself."

Mary was stern. "No you won't," she said, "That's silly."

She was right, of course. In my effort to hang on to normality I was showing my macho. "Well then, I'll wake my neighbor. Actually, it will be quicker."

So I woke John Granville, a good friend in the house next to ours. He came quickly, and we drove to the emergency room in lively conversation as if we were driving to a book party or an art opening. Whatever had happened to my heart, I was not agitating it more. Reliably, Mary Johnson was waiting for us. My journal entry the next day:

> *July 5, 1984*　A whole new episode—the heart—to add to my cancer experience. . . . Got EKG with offbeat pattern, went to intensive care unit to be monitored, called Steve in New York, who got milk train and arrived that morning. . . . Dr. DeCarlo was puzzled, no clear evidence of a heart attack but must make worst-case assumption there was one. Steve in touch with Barondess, who sent his last EKG by jitney. Waiting for analysis of comparative siting and of laboratory blood results tomorrow. . . .
>
> It shows again the vulnerability of my state. Only

eight hours earlier I sent off an upbeat letter to Jen in London ending with my, "Sail on, frail vessel" adjuration to myself. . . . Last night in intensive care I suddenly awoke to ask whether I am in fact taking command, thought everything through, sent for Steve, and we worked out a plan. I could then sleep. Also won my battle with the nurses to sit in a chair a few hours a day. . . . What is striking is the double-volley attack, from cancer *and* heart. The two killers together, a little like the W. S. [Shakespeare] sonnet—

> But in the onset come. Then shall I taste
> At first the very worst of Fortune's might.

But which of the two was "the very worst?" . . . Talked with Mary Ellin [Barrett] today of the episode when Marvin all but died of his second heart attack. . . . She recalled what I had said to her (in my cancer phase): "I have come to terms with my mortality."

It was a pact I had struck with death earlier, in my high need, and I was having to act it out again. One favoring fact was that I had somehow made it to the hospital: the familiar statistic was that at least half the people who die of heart attacks die before the hospital trip or on the way. I reflected that it couldn't have been a particularly lethal onslaught.

I was right, as all three doctors in the end agreed:

> Yesterday the news that it *was* an attack—the series of blood tests and EKGs show it—the second EKG following hard on the first, the second blood test showing the "slightly elevated" enzymes. . . . Today the third series confirms it. . . . A talk with Dr.

DeCarlo and Mary Johnson. DeC. is an efficient, handsome young man, looking like Norman Cousins as I recall him in his 30s. Dr. Mary is magnificent. . . . So now I join the cancer-heart legion! Do I feel depressed? Probably, but I take countermeasures for my subjective mood. The fact is I am a survivor. I have had five close encounters with the Dark Man— lymphoma, lungs (and surgery in both cases), prostate, pneumonia and complications, and now heart. Which leaves me, like a cat, with four more lives to venture.

On the weekend I had a visit from Jerry Barondess, at once internist and cardiologist, with a summer home in the Hamptons:

> Jerry here this A.M. Breezed in with his characteristic brio while I was regaling Steve and his young Mary Ellin [Barrett] with tales of my aberrant life. I recounted to Jerry the onset of the episode and the rest. He examined my heart, read the charts, and came back to say I *had* an attack, but a "minor" one (an "anterior subendocardial infarction"). That it was worse in the pain than the damage. That it had affected not the main heart highways but a small branch. That the blood had to force its way into that clogged branch, producing the lesion, but the trunk and big branches remained unaffected. After 2 weeks at the hospital he sees another two at home, "pretending you have had a heart attack," then slow regaining of a regular life, and I can travel by Sept. and Oct. . . . As for transferring to N.Y. Hospital he is mostly against it: "This is a good little hospital." . . . About

my long-range prospects: "We have learned something from people who live long. The best way to
have a long life is to have a chronic disease." With
that . . . he breezed out. It was Jerry at top form.

I accepted Jerry Barondess's last remark for the professional
blarney it was, intended to ease the self-pity of the afflicted. It
had a paradoxical truth, however, which has stuck with me,
affording a measure of rueful compensation: that chronic illness
carries with it a watchful affirmation of the will to live.

I found that I prefer the intimacy of a small hospital to the
depersonalized big ones. The intensive care unit turned out to
be a self-contained little community, constantly crowded,
where everyone got to know everyone, and the new beds spilled
over into the aisles until old ones could be cleared, and the
nurses and I carried on an affectionate struggle over what I was
allowed to do, and how fast, which always ended in detente.

I was a hospital veteran by now, which enabled me to practice a patterned evasion of the rules, the most innocent form of
law-breaking. Hospitals still carry a residue of the cardiology
model of a decade ago when patients were supposed to be bed-
ridden for days and free of mental as well as physical activity. I
felt in my gut that this was wrong for me. I promoted myself to
a chair early in the game, did my columns and wrote in my
journals, and carried on spirited, sometimes hilarious, conversations with my visiting family and friends. There was much
genuine laughter, except that my sense of the future hurt a bit
when I laughed.

I was holding conversations with myself as well about this
critical organ, the heart, which had sent me an unexpected message to take better notice of it. On the spleen and prostate, both
tumor-ridden, my doctors' verdict had been one of a dispens-
able nuisance, and I came to agree on both scores, adjective and

noun together. My heart was different. Central to my being, I couldn't live without it. Nor had it done anything to offend me. *I* had offended *it* by getting one of my arteries so clogged that the heart couldn't pump enough blood through it without over-taxing and damaging itself. The heart is a good logistical citizen in the polity of the organism, pumping, carrying, delivering our lifeblood—a vital messenger (the Greeks thought) whom the gods provided for us, like their own Hermes. Like Hermes also, deservedly or not, the heart acquired the reputation of being wily and secretive, in fact, something of a thief, going on ma-rauding expeditions, stealing other hearts.

Each age discovers a metaphor for the heart—cosmic sun of the body, mechanical pump, central delivery system, electrical animator—in the image of its own prevailing technology. Our current age has not yet satisfactorily found its own, assigning the dominant neural computer analogy to serve for the brain.

It is hard to contrive a similar contemporary metaphor for the heart, which is ironic, since it has itself been metaphor for so much in us. Its past associations were always positive: with the emotions and passions, with love and commitment, with a be-nign openness to experience, with intuitive insight as against cognitive reasoning, with whatever is central to our lives. One thought of Pascal's great aphorism on the "reasons of the heart" and Tocqueville's on the "habits of the heart."

Metaphor or not, I learned a lesson in medical perspective from a comment made by Vincent Hollander, my Socratic guardian spirit at Mt. Sinai. When he returned from a vacation and found a message to call the Southampton Hospital he feared the worst. "What happened, Max?" he asked. "What are you in intensive care for?"

I told him.

"Oh," he said with evident relief. "Thank God, it's only a heart attack."

I asked why he was grateful to the Deity for so traumatic an event.

His response was a classic. "I was afraid it was a return of one of your cancers, or a new one."

His words jolted me out of my single-vision syndrome. I was focusing on my heart incident and what might come in its wake, forgetting that from the time I acquired my cancers I was fair game. My oncologists at Mt. Sinai knew that a heart attack was a grave event, yet their eye was less on the sparrow of my heart than on the more sinister vulture cells that still had a wide range of targets.

As a new member of the growing Cancer-Heart Legion, I was grateful to Vincent Hollander's effort to set my perspective right. I knew that Jim Holland and Jerry Barondess shared his view. But while medical logic was with them, for me at the moment the danger of a recurring cancer was more distant than the existential fact of living with a precarious heart.

The newcomer in the *dramatis personae* of my life was *angina pectoris,* the tensing of the chest that takes place when the heart's muscle sends a message of needing oxygen because its arterial blood supply is obstructed. You can have a succession of anginas, and put a couple of nitroglycerine wafers under your tongue to deal with them, and survive. But you live in insecurity, never knowing when the heart will suffer unacceptable damage.

In the hospital and out of it, you get to watch for the telltale shortness of breath, the constriction, the sudden body heat and sweating. It could be nothing, or something. The psychic landscape I had experienced as a cancer patient was considerably more rugged: you climbed up craggy rocks and down steep precipices and across terrifying chasms. By contrast my landscape as a heart patient was less dramatic, even a bit dull. But the insecurity of having an "unstable angina" was unremitting.

Fresh out of the hospital, in a talk with my young cardiologist, I asked the usual question: How did things look for the future? His answer was candid. At eighty-one, as I was then, I bore the heavy handicap of age. In case of serious trouble—arterial blockage—a younger man could turn to an angioplasty (the ingenious "balloon" procedure) or even a coronary bypass—double, triple or quadruple, depending on the number of arteries affected. But in my case and at my age, he said gravely, either of them would be too "intrusive," which was a way of saying my heart couldn't take it.

It was less chilling "news" than that of my cancers. I didn't have to face the rigors of surgery, chemotherapy, or radiation, with their sometimes scary statistics of survival. Instead, if things got tough, I faced a blind alley: no exit!

That put the burden on me to keep my arteries lean and clean and give my heart a chance by staying out of trouble. But it also put the burden of vigilance on me.

At the start I carried the burden too heavily. I was careful about everything—stairs, overexertion, lifting and straining. I stopped trying to open or close difficult windows. I had read of anginas that caught the patient unaware, in a sleep that never ended in waking, a thought that sent me on some nights into an anxiety about falling asleep. I never left on any mission, however brief, without a kit which contained a vial of nitroglycerine tablets. I clung to it—and to the twenty-four-hour patch of the same mixture I wore on my chest or arms—as my lifeline. They were my warding-off talismans. I took my prescribed medication every six hours, breaking up my night sleep to do it. My entire ritual was in a sense a mantra that I kept repeating for its warding-off efficacy.

All this may in fact have been prudent survivalism, but it also became an exercise in neurotic invalidism. Behind this fear of anginas (I now see) was the fear of a second, perhaps fatal, heart attack. Much of it was self-induced. No doctor ever lectured me on it. I suspect that for most people with heart problems it comes with the territory of the initial trauma. This may be especially true if the episode follows an earlier life-threatening disease, as was true of the cancer-heart brigade I had joined.

I don't particularly like the kind of person I became for some eighteen months after the attack. I was too fearful, too tied to every daily contingency, too responsive to phantoms in my mind.

My first cancer taught me how to take the stark, calculable prospect of death. The heartbreak of the second cancer was the sense that after the darkness of the pit, and the step-by-step ascent into the light, I was being plunged back in. The heart attack, a less traumatic episode, coming when I felt I had mastered both cancers, stretched the trauma beyond its actual life-threatening dimension. Suddenly I was Sisyphus with his rock. He was the unfortunate condemned by the gods to roll a huge stone uphill without ever getting it to the top, having always to start again from scratch. My fear of the anginas, however based or baseless, now strikes me as a gate I opened to the Adversary, who was not the anginas but fear itself.

It was accentuated by a whole range of symptoms in the first summer (1984) and the following one in 1985, the summer of my discontents. There were pains in the gastrointestinal region that Vincent Hollander followed up by a series of tests, and a pelvic pain that was similarly without result. There was a commotion about a possible cancer of the gum that had Jim Holland stirred up for a while, and which led to a biopsy without results.

The wildest chase of all was the tracking down of a nasty incapacitating, repetitive pain in my right temple that persisted for weeks, despite sedation, and made work and sleep impossible and life dreary. An array of doctors, both at Southampton and Mt Sinai, found no clue to the source until Vincent Hollander and my dentist, Dr. Kenneth Jackier, hit on the answer independently, a malformation of the jaw and teeth (temperomandibular joint syndrome, or TMJ), probably caused by tension.

I have had few symptoms in the past six years to compare with that sustained Time of Troubles for my heart and spirit. I have never adequately resolved what was at the root of it, nor have my doctors. Yet I find a clue of sorts when I ask myself what ended it. Sometimes it is useful to live life backward in order to see what went awry when one lived it forward.

Looking back there was, I think, a period at which my will and life force asserted themselves and I took over the healing of my heart. It was when I said a measured but firm farewell to the thought that at any moment the sword would fall—the angina would become more than an angina—and I would be visited by another heart attack.

There was no one dramatic moment when the change came. It was a convergence of events and of changed attitudes and exploration on my part. I had the first of several talks with Dr. Dean Ornish, a cardiologist in San Francisco, who was on the cutting edge of research on diet and exercise for "reversing" the effects of heart attacks. I now understood that except for the usual pharmaceuticals, my heart infarction wasn't severe enough to require interventions. Besides I was too old for intrusive ones. Thus I had no treatment peg on which to hang my healing. But out of conversations with doctors and friends, and the new literature, and some wayward intuitions, I contrived the regimen of nutrition, walking, gym workouts, work, and controlled environments which was essential to start the slow "reversal" of the arterial blockages. I read Norman Cousins' *The Healing Heart* and found it as inspiriting as it has been for many readers. Finally, I had long talks with Michael, whose basic interest lay in healing approaches to life-threatening diseases. He helped me carry over my affirmative thinking from my cancers to my heart. I had already modified my diet but I now changed it more sharply for my heart, omitting meats, fats, and most dairy products, emphasizing fruits, fish, soups, baked potatoes, and vegetables aplenty.

I was not overly concerned about diet however and carried my vigilance lightly. I was not about to replace an anxiety about anginas with an anxiety about nutrition. What counted, with food as with life, was the pleasure I continued to find in them, undiminished by prudence.

Knowing how much the traditional heart therapy owed to pharmaceuticals, I also sensed the dangers of leaning too heavily on them. So I talked my medications over with Jerry Barondess, who pruned the list to the bare essentials and shifted me from a six- to an eight-hour schedule. It worked, and I felt less drugged and could get an unbroken night's sleep. I was able to slough off my anxieties about medications. I ceased to be an obsessive medicine taker, no longer compulsively clutching my nitroglycerine vial. I don't know just when I banished it, but by the summer of 1986, two years after my heart episode, the negative imagery I had built up was gone.

The world of the imagination is a creative one. When it takes the form of willed imaging, as in the battles I directed between my destructive and healing cancer cells, it can be an auxiliary to recovery. Yet sometimes imaging, unwilled and unwilling, can arise from fears and nourish them. The imagination, instead of serving the therapy, becomes a form of bondage and a blockage to recovery. In *Gestalt* terms it turns the ailment into a long-term center-stage "figure" instead of allowing it to be absorbed into "ground."

The ultimate image is the self-image. It isn't a given; we fashion and refashion it, within the frame of our "can't helps." It is probably the closest we come to being citizens of the realm of self-fulfilling prophecy: what we imagine ourselves to be, in the end we tend to become.

I was now trying to reverse the process, to *un-*become the anxious compulsive, to move in my imagination to my more carefree years when I traveled light, parked my conflicts, and threw away the ticket. I began flying again, to go *somewhere,* after a spell when I felt I had to cancel lectures and interviews and go nowhere for fear of anginas. My seminars were again as full of laughter as they had ever been and—light-hearted once more—I was able to join in.

If I had to fix on a physical symbol for the change, it was walking. In a sense it filled for me the role that laughter played for Norman Cousins in his *Anatomy of an Illness,* not so much the *cause* of my changed mood as its accompaniment and expression. I started my planned walking in Southampton in the late spring of 1986 and continued it into September, adding pace and distance gradually. The road I walked daily ran between the links of the National Golf Club and the inlet of Peconic Bay, to Ram's Island and, when time allowed to the bay itself, a roundtrip of some three and a half miles.

It carried memories for me. It was the course I used to do on a bicycle, summer after summer, battling with whatever tumults my work and life offered. It now became my heart's hegira, at the sun's setting—its tints varying between lemon and orange and rose—and as I walked my route I digested the day's ideas and writing and planned out my work for the morrow. I carried my current workbook with me, and as I watched a little family of swans and the flying geese, I would plot out (in the Yeats phrase) "what was past and passing and to come" in my workbook and my universe.

 During our spells in the city, Jenny and I made a habit of the

East River walkway near our apartment, which the younger
and spryer generation used as a jogging ground. I was lucky to
have the meeting of earth, sky, and water in both settings that
matched a growing serenity within. The title of Milan Kund-
era's *Unbearable Lightness of Being,* which happened to come
out around that time, expressed my mood better than any
words of my own.

From my walking regimen it was a natural progression to
working out in a gym. I began it in California, where the car
culture virtually criminalizes walking. As it happened, Hugh
Hefner, who gives me a second home when I do my California
seminars, added a gym to his home just when I needed it. With
its assemblage of ingenious contrivances for reinvigorating
every muscle and tendon, the gym became for me a kind of Le
Corbusier "machine for living."

So I gradually stepped up the weights for chest, legs, and
back and communed with the stationary bicycle and punching
bag. I always managed to find time for a workout—early morning, late afternoon, sometimes late evening. To ritualize my
physical regimen for my heart and its arterial blood flow was an
added payoff for my structured compulsivity. In time I took my
writing down to the gym, whatever I was working at. For a
couple of hours I alternated physical with mental workouts,
stopping between machines to jot down a phrase or thought as
it came, stopping between sentences to stretch the tensions out
of my system.

All this paid off in unexpected ways, as a journal note attests,
written after one of my semi-annual bone scans in New York,
which are meant to monitor any re-emergence of a cancer.

November 10, 1988   The "nuclear medicine" expert,
Dr. Stanley Goldsmith, who has done my recent bone
scans, called me in for a talk after the scan. Looked

grave, and I wondered what was afoot. Only that my scan shows some remarkable skeletal improvement, a new "vibrant equilibrium." I told him I had been using the noun in my journal notes but had never coupled it with the adjective. If he were "studying it without knowing (me) he would call it the skeleton of a forty-year old." Holy cow and shades of Mahatma Gandhi! He says "we don't understand why this happens, but there it is." . . . I honor his professional humility. But my own guess is that it's the months of workouts with my machines of healing at Hef's. I am tempted to indite a Hymn to the Gym.

I carried over to my California regimen the routine I had formed on my Southampton walks to Peconic Bay. Indeed, I had started something similar during boyhood nights at the century's start in New Haven, when I recited the classic orations to empty streets and sleeping houses on an all-night milk route. It was a dialogue of mind and body in which both are interlocked and each is quickened. I had broached it during the experience with my cancers and lost it for a time as I struggled with my angina fears. I rediscovered it in my walks and gym workouts and my writing, as I sought greater freedom for my arteries and a degree of healing for my heart.

Anyone who gets a dangerous illness is likely to become a watcher of the medical skies, waiting, like John Keats, for a "new planet" to "swim into his ken." In the treatment of illness there is a considerable distance between conventional wisdom and the kind of innovation that stretches the state-of-the-art limits. I would have wished a less punishing drug than the chemotherapies, but that was the state-of-the-art at the time. I was luckier in my prostate cancer because, as I have described, two

Nobel scientists had fought each other over the cutting-edge discovery that rescued me.

I wish a similar discovery had been available in the service of my heart, but it wasn't. There was no one like William Harvey, who charted the entire river system of my heart—great streams, tributaries, and all—which formed its supply-and-support system and its ecology. From Harvey to the medical and surgical elite of today, there is a span of three centuries, to say nothing of the gulf between their respective medical cultures, between the dawning of modern science in the early seventeenth century and our post-modern technology. What they have shared, however, is the sense of the heart as an ingenious mechanism, electrically charged, with a rich chemical context, a thing of intricate beauty in the labyrinthine setting of its arterial network.

A thousand works of literature and art have linked the heart with the mysteries of God and the universe. In the literature and art of religious mysticism, the heart has been an emblem of a compassionate God. In the hyped up imagery of our own media age, caught up in the reporting about heart transplants and artificial hearts, it is now becoming an emblem of the miracles that science and technology can perform.

Both the heart and the brain are indispensable, but while we know the heart can be replaced mechanically—although not for long—the brain cannot. The evidence that the heart may keep beating for a time, even when the brain is dead, led to a new medical-legal definition of death as marked by the ending of brain rather than of heart functioning. This was a defeat for the primacy the heart had long sustained in literature and myth. The brain now displaces it as the criterion and center of life. Yet the very process of displacement is in the service of the heart, since the shift from a legally dead to a living person gives the transplant a moral validation.

Emerson wrote that he was the possessor of "Shakespeare's

heart and Plato's brain." In the same sense I feel myself the inheritor of Harvey's vision and of the labor and insights of a whole succession of workers in cardiovascular knowledge who came after him. The fact that so few of us know the names and lives of those to whom we are indebted is a sign of how we have come to take for granted what we now call the medical establishment. It is better called the medical culture, since it goes far beyond our existing establishment, which it is constantly displacing.

In our own day we have learned that the heart, brain, and arterial and vascular systems form a force field, both of functioning and vulnerability. We are creating a democracy of illness, and with it a willed search for health. Out of it has come a new elite of cardiac surgeons who have achieved stardom in the medical performing arts and have an impressive mastery of their mystery. Yet, given the upheavals of knowledge and technology that brought them their renown, we must ask what insights and technologies still to come will make them an artifact of a dimly remembered past.

Would I, if a clogged artery or some other unhappiness hit me, deliver myself even at my age into their well-trained hands? In a crisis, if no other recourse were viable, I would find a surgeon who still had the edge of wonder in him. I would be serene about his doing whatever the affected artery needed and stitching me up again, and I would remember him as the shepherd who led me into a green pasture when I could graze nowhere else and restored my functioning and my soul.

The theatrical adventures in heart transplants and artificial hearts are more daring forays into the unknown. They test the fringes of information-age medicine as the art of the impossible. Intellectually I feel drawn to such ventures for their Promethean boldness in stealing fire from the ruling gods. They are a form of assertion of life, even if by proxy.

They push us all into hard thinking about the problem of
limits. Would I, at my unlikely age, agree to a heart transplant
as a last desperate measure?

One could write an essay on whether the continued expan-
sion of the boundaries of the artificial is a legitimate expression
of the healing process or an invasion of the province of God and
nature. The Greek myth of Daedalus and his son Icarus has
usually been taken as an instance of man's technological arro-
gance: Flying too near the sun on wings his father had fash-
ioned, Icarus plunged to a sea death. But I go with James Joyce
when he calls Daedalus the "fabulous artificer" and names his
hero for him. The Daedalean vision, risks and all, is part of
what the creative encounter was about, for the Greeks as for us,
in science and inventiveness. The risks go with the territory of
living.

I am not worried about the "artificial" as against the "natural," nor do I charge society and its technology with corrupting
"natural man." Freud suffered from cancer of the mouth, and
the prosthesis for it was bungled, yet he was himself still doctor
enough to see that "the future belongs to prosthetic man."

I like my heart, battered as it is. But if my doctors were to tell
me that it is pretty much done for, and offer me a stranger's
heart in its place, I would try to make the alien heart feel at
home for as long as our destiny together dictated. If there were
no recourse but an artificial heart, I would embrace it and say,
"Pump away, oh Fabulous Artificer, while it is day, for the
night comes when no heart can pump."

10. The Upward Spiral: The Doctor Within the Patient

Each patient carries his own doctor inside him. . . . We are at our best when we give the doctor who resides within each patient a chance to work.

— Albert Schweitzer

Let us give Nature a chance; she knows her business better than we do.

— Michel Montaigne, *Essays*

The world belongs to me because I understand it.

— Honoré de Balzac

I AM, AS I WRITE, in the midst of a vigorous, sustained healing phase. I never expected a "cure" for either of my cancers or for my heart infarction, since "cure" implies a restoration of some status quo in the golden past. It goes against the grain of what we know about how the organism works. When Dr. Dean Ornish speaks of "reversibility" after or before a heart attack, I like the term better than "cure." It means only that a downward spiral can be converted to an upward spiral. Instead of a theory of the mind–body connection, I want to relate how the upward spiral of healing operated in my own case. Perhaps it has a parallel in the experience of others.

By "healing" I mean the reaching for a new balance within ourselves and with our society, environments, and relationships, all of which an illness throws off balance. From the start I refused to make a choice between two modalities of healing, the traditional one, which stresses the effect of medical interventions by doctors, chemicals, and pharmaceuticals, and the holistic one, which sees the patient as more than the sum of the parts into which the specialist splits him and stresses the powers of his mind and will.

In an area as tangled as health, it is wise to resist either/or dichotomies and seek instead the principle of polarities. On the surface we speak of opposing entities: love–hate, war–peace, hawk–dove, friend–enemy, simplicity–complexity. But as we explore them, the unyielding dichotomies turn into polar fields which fuse elements of both. If it is true of life and death in their interaction and containment of each other, why should it not be true also of the polar modalities of healing, where we can acknowledge both the efficacy of interventions from without and the power of mind and spirit within?

In this setting the best role for the doctor is to provide the experience and judgment that will enable these two healing processes to engage each other—interventions and will. It would be wrong to assign only the first to the doctor. Yet in our bureau-cratic medical culture the doctor's role of guide through the specialist maze, which has become his accepted one, has all but swallowed his earlier function as a shaman, endowed with a touch of magic.

The cultural anthropologists, writing about magic, medicine, and myth among primitive cultures, tell us of the belief in the capacity of the shaman to release the self-healing powers of the sick and restore their peace of body and soul. In modern usage we refer to the triggering of the action of the immune system in its links with the brain and neural systems. This *shaman effect* took on a personal meaning for me, offering a clue to the mys-tery of healing and self-healing.

There are still authentic doctors, young and old, who retain their healing touch and whose authority shines through, evok-ing a responsive chord of life-affirming self-belief in the patient. I can bear witness to this in instances of my own experience with my doctors. I wish it were true of more doctors, in the service of more patients.

Why isn't it? Part of the key may lie in the freezing of the roles of both doctor and patient, the doctor's in presenting his diagnoses and therapies from on high, the patient's in accepting them passively. Whatever interaction takes place is routine. Neither touches nor releases a spring of affirmation in the other. The entire model tilts toward the rigid.

Even if I didn't have a life stake in exploring this scenario I would still be drawn to it as an intellectual problem. We are all today reaching out for some hypothesis of healing which carries with it a probing of mysteries beyond our present grasp. At this safe distance I might now, wryly, see the years of illness as a form of field work, and the energies devoted to self-healing as my personal testing ground of the mind–body connection.

The problem of the doctor–patient relation in healing is not easily resolved. I argued it out with myself in several September 1987 journal entries:

> There can be no denying the shaman effect on healing, in whatever culture—including our own. Freud recognized it, and it became part of the mental therapy tradition, in the form of "transference." It exists also in other (nonmental) therapies, where the doctor's one-on-one role in the dialogue with the patient is more tenuous. Here a question sticks out awkwardly: how invoke and use the shaman effect when the doctor's authority is so widely questioned?

> There is a clue here, if not quite an answer. We think of doctors less as *healing* than as simply *treating* us. Whether it is chemotherapies, surgeries, radiation, or other interventions, treatment has become largely impersonal and routinized, with a bewildering array of people involved in it. The patient must still trust the doctor in the sense of believing he is competent and knows what he is doing. But that's a long way from a healing relationship. . . . Unlike treatment, healing involves a patient open and interactive with the doctor. In all cultures the shaman has been part of a self-healing process by the belief and trust he inspires. In traditional societies, where change is slow, authority prime and potent, and the individual counts for less than kin and tribe, the shaman practices his sorcery, and the magus exerts his magic, by releasing the self-healing strength of the patient.

> In our highly individualist society, where we have largely abandoned collective belief, and total trust in

doctors is hard to come by, we have moved far from the shaman model. Yet strikingly the need (and even yearning) for the shaman effect—for someone who will trigger the self-healing resources of the patient—is surfacing even more strongly. Not all doctors have the shaman element in them. I am lucky to have had several to work with me in my need. There are many doctors—and many nondoctors—who inspire the trust needed for this self-healing. In their absence the patient must find a way of releasing it within himself. The fact that many are doing it now is the glory of the patient's revolution within the larger selfhood revolution.

I felt this was leading in the right direction, but I was not home yet. I had to argue out a final objection in my meditative journal entry:

Can I have it both ways—placing the patient at the center of the healing constellation, yet also giving so much emphasis to the shaman in the doctor? . . . Yes, in fact it rounds out the scenario. While the doctor provides the options and skills, it is the patient who must have within him the self-healing potential which a good doctor can release. While the doctor invests a segment of his selfhood in one patient after another, the patient must invest all his selfhood. . . . Yet each must also surrender a portion of his selfhood to the other. The patient finds a way to trust the judgments and intuitions of the doctor of his final choice. The doctor finds a way to release the self-healing dynamic of the patient. Each stoops to conquer, for a joint victory. Each enables the other to exercise his functions to the full, and out of the fusion comes healing.

These reflections may suggest why every era has invested its life-threatening diseases with symbolic significance. They cut close to our involvement with the elementals of life and death. Whenever any of these diseases touched public policy, my experience with illness was bound to color my views, as a commentator, about what was happening in the medical-political world outside.

If contingency is the tyrant, I feel, the subjective will is the rebel to overthrow him, or at least make him become a democratic king, accountable to us. The struggle against illness is part of a wider struggle for the freedom and autonomy of the individual, by little bands of people acting together, as always in history. We create the tyrannies we must strive against—the establishments and their rigidities, the false gods and their idol images.

At one point a journal note picked up this thinking, with some personal feeling:

> *November 15, 1987* . . . The reality is that patients are lining up to wait for drugs difficult of access, and for experimental protocols hard to get into. . . .
>
> I came to identify strongly with them. During my dark years I scanned the literature for news of anything that could bend the odds for me. But it wasn't the doctor we all wanted: it was the intervention of the drug, and the doctor—whether a commercial researcher or a government functionary—came with it. . . . In most cases the drug is critical, particularly when speed in getting in on the experimental protocol . . . is a matter of life and death. I know that if I had not got in on Buserelin I would not today have breath or balls.

I was not heedful of the decorous word, but the passion that broke through as I wrote is still relevant to what is happening in medical politics, as witness a later journal entry:

> *February 29, 1988*   I count myself a medical Populist. I want as many people as possible to get in on the risky winged thing that brings hope to people who are starved of hope. I get angry at the rigid review panels of doctors, and the routineer bureaucrats in Washington who form a bottleneck which keeps the drug from being available during scary months and years. I get angrier when they say they are doing it in the name of science and for the good of the patients. I want to blast the bottleneck—and them with it. Who are they to keep patients, all of us, from taking what risks we are determined to take, in the cause of life and its possibilities? To be human is to be a risk taker. No one can substitute his role playing for my autonomy when my life is the stakes. . . . My medical Populism reaches deeper than the political Populism, which responds to the needs of the disaffected. This Populism, in the universe of the ill, responds to the needs of the risk takers, trying to salvage their lives.

I have been disheartened by the failure of the political culture to take up the cause of the people as sufferers, against the medical and governmental bureaucracies. Those fighting for autonomy of choice, and freedom of access, having peered into the heart of darkness, have seen enough to forgo parochial perspectives and direct the focus of life itself.

This gives a new meaning for me to Albert Schweitzer's "reverence for life," which I interpret as reverence for the life force within the humblest people. Working at Lambarene, in Africa, his knowledge of medical procedures and technology was limited. But "my life is my argument," he said repeatedly, and what he lived and argued for—access to medical help for everyone and entry thereby for the healer within us all—is still worth arguing and living for.

I don't know how much of my present state is owed to my doctors, medications, and family, how much to my own often blundering efforts of the self-observing and self-healing will. Yet the reality as I write is that ten and eight years after my respective tumors, my cancer-scarred lymph glands and prostate are still within me, causing little trouble. Six years after my heart attack, I have my heart, still pumping blood through tolerably clear arteries. My riddled organs and I have learned to get along together in a working pact. Following our tumultuous wars I have reached a separate peace with each, however unstable a peace with a wild cell or a cloggable artery may be.

I add two entries from my journal during my illness. One was written several weeks after I turned eighty-two:

> *January 11, 1984* I have a theory that coming into command of my illness has made me more capable of coming into command of my life. . . . For the first time since my illness I feel I may well get to the end of my 80's, which is equivalent to saying I feel immortal!

Ironically, after this vaunting bit and some setbacks that followed it, my journal records another entry:

> *October 3, 1984* I may stumble into darkness suddenly. But death will catch me in motion . . . still invested with the *mysterium tremendum* of life, death, and love, of God and the cosmos—which at this point is the only way I know of transcending death.

11. Aging: The Last Voyage

And so, from hour to hour we ripe and ripe,
And then from hour to hour we rot and rot,
And thereby hangs a tale.

— William Shakespeare, *As You Like It*

An aged man is but a paltry thing,
A tattered coat upon a stick, unless
Soul clap its hands and sing, and louder sing
For every tatter in its mortal dress. . . .

— William Butler Yeats, *Sailing to Byzantium*

Nothing can be meaner than the anxiety to live on, to live on
anyhow and in any shape; a spirit with any honor is not willing to
live except in its own way, and a spirit with any wisdom is not
over-eager to live at all.

— George Santayana, *Winds of Doctrine*

The older I grow the more impressed I am by the frailty and
uncertainty of our understanding, and all the more I take recourse
to the simplicity of immediate experience so as not to lose contact
with the essentials, namely, the dominants which rule human
existence throughout the milleniums.

— C. G. Jung, at eighty-five

H OW CAN I LEAVE THIS MEMOIR of my illness without giving an account of the aging process that went with it?
In the order of things, starting with the darkness, God
created the Heavens and the Earth, then man and woman and
their health, their illness, their prime and aging—before the
final darkness which rounds out the cycle.

All through my sequence of maladies and healings I had also
to cope with the fact of growing old. It was a case of morbidity
and mortality jostling for precedence to decide which would
overcome the other in their unseemly eagerness to hasten me to
the terminal point. Aging is what, in its wisdom or mischief,
time does to the organism, making it progressively dysfunc-
tional, using it up until it is too worn out to go on. I have to add
that for a period before its ending, time evokes also its riper
qualities.

"That is no country for old men," wrote Yeats, with Ireland
as his setting but with the West as his larger target. Even as it
has become an aging society, America in particular still has its
cult of youth. Throughout my writing and teaching I stormed
against this cult and its disdain for maturity and age, yet I did it
in my classes, where I liked being surrounded by the young. I
have, I fear, been boastful about my age, counting it the insignia
of experience. In the battle over whether we should spend or
conserve our energies, I sided with the spenders. Life was there
to be lived to the full. I spent myself in every direction.

In time I paid for it. I see now that my illness was part of
living itself. So is my aging. I have tried to nourish as few illusions about aging as about illness. I see the travail of aging as
the squalors which our creatureliness in time brings with it.
Unless we face them, we have not paid the entry fee for the
other aspect of aging—its satisfactions and joys. Like the god of
war, aging is Janus-faced, with a double presence.

People in primitive societies don't keep track of aging by

counting the years. They depend on collective memory of events that stand out in tribal history, and on rites of passage as they go through life. For modern man the counting syndrome is obsessive.

There are three simultaneous aging phases: *calendar* aging, largely a social construction with society doing the counting; *organismic* aging, whose pace varies with every individual but whose underlying facticity cannot be denied by any; and *subjective* aging, where the mind filters, tempers, or aggravates what the body presents to it.

We are lucky if we can ignore the first, and the second won't let itself be ignored. I humored the signs of my aging organism. After all, I did in time get hearing aids fitted. But it is in the third—our subjective sense of how old or young we are—where we may get a chance to affect in some measure the rigors of a stern evolutionary process.

If aging is the movement of the organism toward dissolution, as I have suggested, it is inherent in life itself. More strictly, it is the phase of the life process in which the balance gradually shifts, and what is vulnerable in the organism begins to encroach upon what is functionally operative.

This happens to each of us at an uneven pace, depending on the system involved: the deterioration of motor skills tends to come early, that of memory and some other mental faculties later. But early or late, at a different pace, with a different intensity, this encroachment happens to all.

I had not taken my aging seriously until I collided with its reality during my illness, when I had to ask what was due to illness and what to aging, and found few answers. All through my seventies I had led an active life in everything that counted for me, rationalized my physical shortfalls, and felt pretty cocky about moving toward my eighties with a self-image that carried few scars. In my innocence, I was thus quite unprepared for the experience of being sick and old together.

In my late seventies a friend who was a documentary film-maker, Robin Lehman, came out to Southampton to include me in a film he was shooting. He called it *Forever Young,* and it also starred a half-dozen other specimens from his aging butter-fly collection. I spouted some philosophy about love and work, rode a bike jauntily toward the camera, and enacted the closing scene by walking across the ocean dunes toward the sunset, hand in hand with a little girl. It was the purest corn and I felt a twinge at the playacting in it—but I loved it, perhaps because I felt genuinely a seamlessness between my mid-years and late years.

About the same time, on the eve of my first cancer, I did a couple of TV interviews with Bill Moyers, two hours of conver-sation on presidential history and politics with a master crafts-man. I enjoyed them. After my cancer had set in, and at a bleak point of my chemotherapy, there was an unexpected repeat of the show, which Jenny and I happened to catch. It was a painful experience to see my precancer image and to feel the change. The seamlessness I have mentioned had been ripped away by my illness. For the first time it struck me fully that illness and aging bring a true break with the past. They are an unholy alliance, more powerful together than either apart.

One way I came to confront my aging was to carry on a running dialogue with it in my journals:

April 5, 1988 "The gods have become diseases," wrote Jung. Since aging is a disease of sorts, how about a god of aging? The Greeks had Chronos to represent Time. Note that he ate his children (the great Goya painting at the Prado, in Madrid) as Time eats us whom it has begotten. It is a savage painting but expresses the feeling we all have at the enormity of what Time does to us.

I wrote this entry on a New York City bus, on my way to visit a doctor. Jenny reminds me now that Chronos ate his children to balk the prediction that they would kill him. Which is doubtless so, but it doesn't affect the truth of Time's ravages. As my journal note continues, the reference to Yeats is to his poem, "Sailing to Byzantine," some of whose lines form an epigraph at the start of this chapter:

Here am I on a bus, a "tattered coat upon a stick," as Yeats had it—with a continuing cough, and a crick in my neck that won't go away, my bloodshot eyes moving toward cataracts, my hearing all but gone were it not for prosthetic aids, my prosthetic bridges also there to help me chew, my skin variegated and splotched like an old frog in a pond. Here am I, creaking as I bend down to pick up something, weaving a bit as I walk, half-numb in my feet, racked by alternating sweats and shivers, dependent for life on regular doses of nitroglycerine and my daily injection of the analog of the extract from a sheep's or pig's brain. Here am I, forced to stay in my favoring environments, strapped into them when I would wish to be roaming the continents with Jenny as we used to do when I was younger. . . . Yet here am I also, not just "happy" but joyful at being alive, with family and friends, with all the faculties that count most, with mind and passions and imagination I hope undimmed, loving and loved to my heart's satiety, thinking, teaching, writing my brains out.

Yeats wrote his poems about old age in his late sixties and early seventies, which we now see as the early aging phase, but he wrote with an imagination fevered by the intense consciousness of growing old. Note how he moved on to the splendid *unless:*

> ... unless
> soul clap its hands and sing, and louder sing
> For every tatter in its mortal dress.

It is Soul that counts, especially in aging, Soul clapping its hands and singing.

As the entries that follow suggest, I used my journals as a ledge to stand on, for whatever hand clapping and singing I could manage. I start with an extended journal entry at Bolinas, where Jenny and I visited with Michael during one of the cancer retreats over which he presides, at Commonweal:

> *October 22, 1987*   I walk through a primeval forest of rotting pines and oaks, and come out suddenly into the sunlight, with the beach of the Pacific stretching in a rough arc below me, precipitously. . . . What is this aging? I am on the threshold of 85, with a still vibrant life force.
>
> Five years from now, at 90, a decade from now at 95, if I am still I, what will be different in me? Will there be a steady diminution of energy, a thinning out of zest, a deadening of the fierceness of joy I now feel? And how will it come about? Will it be by a series of organismic "events," no one of them substantial in itself, but together mounting insidiously to a sense of disability, until the final event (from within or without) that my weakened heart cannot withstand?

I was putting questions to age with an insistence induced by the sense of the decaying trees and the springing up of flowers at their base, and the enduring stretch of ocean below. I continued with a troubling aspect of my questions on aging:

> Is aging itself a disease that establishes a commonality of affliction among us all? If it is, why can't I fight it with the help of the immune system and the self-healing force it releases, as I have done in part with my cancers and my heart? . . . Perhaps one answer is that we never fully "recover" from any illness, at whatever age—that each new equilibrium leaves our functioning impaired and our resistance to the next illness weakened. In that sense we are aging and indeed dying from the moment of our birth. In the later years there is an acceleration of both, not arithmetically but exponentially. . . . If aging is regressive, as seems all too clear, it is a regression "punctuated" (as in the theories of evolution) by creative leaps of adaptation. I call them "creative" in the sense that the organism seems capable at times of salvaging, and even inventing, resourceful ways of pursuing its deepest purposes—of research and knowledge, of organizing and managing, painting, music, and the arts of governing.

I concluded the meditative soliloquy with some definitions to help me see aging whole:

> I don't see how, even in our most optimistic mood, we can refuse to define aging as the progressively dysfunctional element in the organism's journey through life, which leaves it ever more vulnerable to the impact of illness and of other disorders and disorienta-

tions. Yet neither do I see how, in our darkest mood, we can refuse to include in the definition what is now established beyond doubt—that there is a creativity in every age which may sustain us until journey's end.

In 1957, in *America as a Civilization,* a book on American life and thought, I included a section on "the middle and end of the journey" as part of the life cycle. Thirty years later, in an Afterword, I noted that "one of the prime aspects of the new America is that an aging revolution is taking place within a larger revolution—that of the social perception of the entire life-journey, and its self-management in the adult stages." More than anything, my coping with illness and aging made me feel part of that selfhood revolution.

It led me to break a few lances in the battle against a stereotyped view of aging which showed up, surprisingly, even in so resourceful a mind as B. F. Skinner's. When he told psychologists in convention that aging is a time when we can no longer "think coherently, logically, or, in particular, creatively," I wrote my own responding credo of aging:

> *September 1, 1982*   I believe years count less than the health of the mind. Diseases come with the territory of life, and they come more closely clustered in the later stages. But some people are fogies when they are young, and others are young in spirit while old in years. . . . I believe it is time to get rid of the cult of youth that has distorted our perceptions of ourselves. What has plagued the aging has been not their years but the image in society that those years should mean a fateful diminution of work, play, sexuality, love, action, passion, imagination, creativity, life hungers, life satisfactions. . . . I believe that each stage has its own kind of creativity. The later stages have fewer undam-

aged brain cells and neural synapses to call on, hence the memory problem. But in turn these stages have the experience of the whole life journey to serve as a perspective. Time becomes not only destroyer but preserver. . . .

Skinner says it is harder at his age to "think big thoughts," that he has to use a rigid outline in his writing to keep from "senile nattering and inconsistencies and repetition." Yet the history of thought and the arts is replete with grand conceptions that have come late in life rather than earlier. The need for "rigid" frames may be Skinner's problem, not a universal one. Rigidity is more likely to come with character structure than with age.

We have been through the grueling battles of casting the devils of stereotyping out of religion, race, and gender. But the aging revolution cuts across all these, involves us all, and may prove to be the most lasting of all.

Too many life-course thinkers—Jung was a notable exception—got caught on the spike of aging and let some of the most fruitful years pass by with hardly a nod. One could understand this in Skinner, a stern behaviorist who disbelieved in anything that smacked of subjectivism. But I felt it important, while asserting the aging revolution, to recognize the stirring changes taking place in the consciousness of Western societies, and redraw the lines of division in order to celebrate the last half of the journey.

In the 1980s, I argued, the cultural realities of modern life have stretched young manhood and womanhood through the thirties and well into their later forties, the midpoint of life. As for the rest of the journey, I see early middle age as reaching

through the fifties into the early sixties, and later middle age—
still vigorous and generative—through the sixties into the early
seventies. For the last two stages I quote from a piece I wrote at
the time:

We are shaping a new category of the young old, from the early 70's to
the mid-80's. Their organisms tell them they are aging but in many—
perhaps most—cases their minds tell them they are still young. It is a
scrappy age for scrappy people. . . . Finally there are the older old,
from the mid-80's to 100 and beyond. They have seen and experienced
everything, yet—with all their ordeals—every year is precious. They
are explorers in uncharted seas, and when I join them I shall call the
group (in Henry V's phrase, addressing his battle commanders) "We
few, we happy few, we band of brothers."

I wrote this at eighty-two, in the midst of my illness battles.
Now I feel part of that band, with some sense of triumph over
obstacles but also of anticipation. Despite a playful note in my
aging schema, underneath it I was wrestling in dead earnest
with the question of dynamics—the *how.* How does it happen
that, in the midst of aging, we hold tenaciously to the life force
which we associate with youth, even though we know that the
outcome is never in doubt?

I found a clue of sorts in Ashley Montagu's *Growing Young,*
a history of the curious concept of *neoteny*—the extension of
the child form, with its openness and playfulness, into maturity.
There is a Rousseau-like sadness in the whole perspective: man
is born free, flexible, loving, with all the characteristics of the
child, yet everywhere he is caught in the chains of the "grown-
ups," who move him toward being rigid, solemn, aggressive,
specialized. It is, says Montagu, society that ages him, not his
biological destiny, which means him to retain his youthful traits
and shed them only at a slow, developmental pace. What Montagu presents is a deterioration story, starting early from the
time when society urges the child not to grow but to *grow up.*

This is an ingenious, if somewhat quirky idea. But it puts too great stress on society as villain and too high a valuation on youthfulness in itself. Our culture, youth-entranced, needs a counterweight to our nostalgia for youth, not a reinforcement of it. I was not seduced by the idea of turning my later years into a second childhood.

I found a different clue in Gerald Heard's learned and neglected classic, *The Five Ages of Man,* which traces the history of human consciousness through five stages and sees them repeated in the life history of the individual. The last stage in the individual human life correlates with the last phase of the collective story of man. Heard calls that stage, the aging one, a "second maturity."

It made more sense to me than a second childhood: the first maturity, of adulthood, will not be shed in aging but transcended. It is vain, in a double sense, either to regress to a youth we must outgrow or to try to retain it when the fact is that life is a moving thing. It is better to see the physical ordeals of aging as the very real price we pay for the chance to move on, in mind and spirit, to a maturity in some ways deeper and more serene than the initial one in the "prime" of life.

When Erik and Joan Erikson, in their mid-eighties, offered a reprise of their famous original model of the stages of the "life cycle," they elaborated a dimension that had been only tacit some forty years earlier: "recapitulation." The "virtue" or "lesson" with which the life struggle at each stage is resolved is picked up by the next. Then old age recapitulates them all, from infancy and youth on, and seeks to integrate them as it fends off the despairs of aging. What results is "wisdom."

I am less confident than the Eriksons about the "wisdom" which they posit at life's closing stage. The danger of the earlier Erikson view lay in portraying the aging phase as an inevitable winding-down: the strength of the later view is that it sees all the preceding stages as preparation for the last and integrative stage, giving the old a selective usable past on which to build.

Whatever the frame each of us prefers, of the ages and stages of aging, abstractly, we are drawn to it by the experience of some vivid personal imagery. The nature of mine will be evident from a journal note:

> June 12, 1988   In imagining my own aging I have the Old Testament patriarchs in mind—Abraham, Isaac, Jacob, David, Solomon. Some of them, we know from the narrative, were cruel and arbitrary. But as a line of succession they were also fecund, generative, intent on giving the children a strong family frame, to grow them up in the knowledge not only of how to rule a kingdom but how to rule themselves and their lives. . . . I was granted three daughters, then three sons. It wasn't until the second brood were growing up that I began to envisage my aging years. Watching them I not only conflated their experiences with my own at their age but I made a leap forward into the time when I could no longer have that young life-stage to integrate with my own. . . . I was 54 when my last-born, Adam, entered life. I knew I would be in my 70's when he entered college and in 80's when he began his career. He was the last of my children but the first to have a grandfather for father. If there was to be a rounding out of a life cycle for me it would have to be in my 80's.

I continue to be, I confess, shamelessly patriarchal. I love the occasions of the gathering of the clan, kin as well as kith, when the authority that family once had in America can be reclaimed, and the place of deference that aging parents had can be restored. There is no masculinism here. Jenny at seventy-six is just as much a matriarch as I am a patriarch. Nor do children and grandchildren blot out their egos in the presence of the old: they are in lively evidence.

Yet the prevailing note is of an extended family, one that is still a polity where the center—of lived experience—must hold if the lessons life teaches are not to fall apart. It is in such a context that a "second maturity," for women and men alike, becomes a second generativity.

The imagination of aging, the shaping of images of its nature and therefore of our own aging years, starts with our first sense of the strange creatures around us who are deemed "old." It is a jumble of shifting images, some benign, some frightening. We don't apply them seriously to ourselves until the threat they convey draws close. Then all our coping mechanisms come into play.

Aging is a stage of life, death a finality. The fear of death is the fear of the unknown as well as the terminal. The fear of aging is the fear of the all too well known. Both prod us into activity. Along with the maladies in its wake, aging forms our early warning system of the approach of death. The fear of death spurs us to invent energies and busyness that will mask its terror from us. The fear of aging—limiting the compass of our lives, diminishing the time that still remains for fruitful functioning—spurs us to fall back and reinvent ourselves, to savor more fully the life that remains. This means to reimagine who and where we are, what we want of the rest of our lives, what we can whittle away as inessential, what becomes central.

To cope with a life-threatening illness at any time, and succeed in overcoming it, has to be in itself a life-changing experience. To be close to death "powerfully concentrates a man's mind," as Dr. Johnson put it. When the illness comes late in life, it adds a touch at once of pathos and piquancy. The pathos is that so few years remain for living with the renewed depth you have achieved. The piquancy is that you are spurred even more to rethink life, to reinvent self, to ask the embracing question: What shall I do with the rest of my life?

Back in the late 1950s and the 1960s, the experts were saying that old age was a time for a man or woman to "disengage"—to mute their intensities, diminish the life-roles they had played, in short, to prepare for death.

When I dug up this literature in the 1980s, having been struck by illness and the realities of aging, its full absurdity became clear. Who were these savants of aging to tell me to disengage at the very moment when I felt the fire of battle, like Nelson at Trafalgar? Who were they to tell me to prepare for death, when death was exactly the adversary I had to confront and somehow outwit? Even before physical death, I was being asked to accept the death of nerve and verve and the will to prevail.

So instead of disengaging I re-engaged with life and death. While once I treated time as if it didn't exist, I am now conscious of the limits it sets. Exactly because time is so grudging to me I can't remain indifferent to it. I must do much with the little space it gives me.

However much I valued continuity, I had no intention of outliving myself by repeating my old life patterns. It made little sense to me to follow Emerson's injunction about aging: to "draw in sail" and pay homage to the "god of limits." True, I got rid of irrelevancies and paid less attention to the "mice" that nibble at us and at our time. True also, I had to accept the physical limits my organism set. I could no longer run and had to walk at a somewhat slower pace, but walk I did. I cut down on my trips to Europe and my former winter jaunts: in fact, "vacations" ceased to have much meaning when work had become a way of staving off the night, and every day a renewal.

I had to recognize the reality principle, yet aging and death as realities were too elusive to be ensnared in the logic trap. So I turned increasingly to narrative, including the narrative of my own crisis experience. I turned also to image, metaphor, and myth, which are the stuff of poetry and tales. I came to understand why the best insights into the experience of old age and approaching death come not from the scientists or doctors but from poets like Tennyson, Hardy, Yeats, D. H. Lawrence.

It was the Tithonus myth that caught my imagination, Tithonus, the beautiful young man to whom the dawn goddess, Aurora, granted the gift of immortality but failed to accompany it with the gift of eternal youth. Tennyson's poem, "Tithonus," takes the form of a lament to the goddess:

> The woods decay, the woods decay and fall, . . .
> And after many a summer dies the swan.
> Me only cruel immortality
> Consumes; I wither slowly in thine arms . . .

Aging is part of mortality, which, with all its ravages, is better than an immortality that denies the human.

In our century Aldous Huxley picked up the Tithonus theme from Tennyson in a novel, *After Many a Summer Dies the Swan,* about the Faustian effort of a Hearst-like Californian, with the help of cutting-edge science, to purchase an unlimited life by his money and power. What it adds up to is that aging has terrors greater than dying. It isn't longer life in itself we desire but life on functional terms, without the intolerable ravages of old age.

It was in Alex Comfort's treatise, *The Biology of Senescence,* that I came up against the harsh limits that the evolutionary cycles place on the "maximum life span potential" of man, along with other creatures of the natural universe. Another journal note:

> Adam at dinner, discoursing on the shoptalk at his molecular biology lab on aging, about the compara-

tive longevity limits that various species can't break through. It is a limit true for any species, one that we have broken our minds against, like waves against a rocky shore: I am not speaking of overcoming death but of prolonging the life of the species set by whatever macro-standard of nature and evolution. I see humans using their intelligence to improve the functioning of human life and extend it as close as possible to the limits of its potential. . . . By whatever means this gets done, I want to get in on the doing. If it takes prosthetic technology, why not? To extend the functional life—a life with meaning—is what counts.

In the winter of my life, which by its integrative quality contains residues of all three earlier seasons, I assert the joys that come with the season, just as I endure its pesky trials. I think more about aging than I did when I was not married to it as a true love. It reaches into my consciousness and becomes a reference point for much else—more for perspective, I trust, than for self-pity.

Again a journal entry may say it with more immediacy:

During the time I write this I have been ineluctably aging. If the thought had occurred to me during the mid-forties to mid-fifties, when I was writing my *America* book, I would have rejected it contemptuously. After all, it was my "prime of life," wasn't it? You don't "age," do you, in your prime, any more than you age as an adolescent, infant, fetus? At those points you "ripe and ripe," as Shakespeare had it. When do you start to "rot and rot?" When does maturity end and decay begin? . . . The physicists speak of a "critical mass," when the ingredients reach a point which only a change of phase can resolve. This happens in the aging phase. All the adjectives we use for what precedes it carry the sense of *budding, growing, ripening,* while those we use for what follows are *decaying, deteriorative,* even *degenerative.* . . . It is true as well in nature and history. Daniel Levinson calls his version of the life cycle the "seasons of a man's life." Oswald Spengler wrote of the "Spring" and "Summer" in the life history of some great ganglion of a people, when they enjoyed a ripening "culture," and he wrote of the "Autumn" and "Winter" when they dried up and rigidified into a late "civilization." . . .

While the leaf on the tree and the early culture phase of a civilization may grow sere and die, the tree renews itself for another round, as do many civilizations. "So careless of the single life, so careful of the race," wrote Tennyson of evolution. Yet with all my vauntings and passions and prides I am a leaf, not a tree. I am a single life, not a race. The sheer facticity of it is that I am decaying to death, just as the individual reed is. Yet though my strength is only that of the reed I am, in Pascal's phrase, a "thinking reed." Hence both the pathos and glory of it.

With the new medical technology we cannot escape thinking about the province of the state in setting terminal limits to life for the old. In order to ration its resources, writes Daniel Callahan, ethicist, in his *Setting Limits* (1987), society must set priorities for the use of technology and medical services. Instead of lavishing them on protracting the life span of the very old and the very sick, he argues, we should use them instead for the "children of the poor."

To use expensive technology in order to keep a vegetable existence going is, I agree, absurd. But if the technology is in place, and the conscious and rational will to live is there, who possesses the moral authority to say who shall have its use and who not? There are clearly cases, at whatever age, where sustaining life artificially makes no moral sense. But if it is a life capable of functioning and the individual and family are agreed, chronological age cannot be a cut-off point. It carries the utilitarian philosophy to the point where it is no longer a moral philosophy. It would substitute a mechanistic view for an organismic one.

We need not be defensive about the autonomy of individual choice. Just as I am a medical populist when it comes to taking risks in gaining access to experimental procedures, so I am an old-age populist when someone old and sick is determined to fight for life. The lasting civilizations have had a regard for age, and for the webbing of cohesion on which that regard was based.

In the 1960s we talked about the "generation gap" and feared a generational war. It started but didn't last. Youth rebellions rise and subside with the tides of politics and values. The awareness of the aging is a mounting existential force. One reason why the generational gap was short-lived may have been the sense of emptiness it left when the young were no longer nourished by familial closeness.

Robert Nisbet argues that elderly pressure groups will trigger a generational class war since it is the young who will bear the burden of paying for the entitlements of the old. There are few young who do not have the care of older family members on their minds. Moreover, the imagination of aging may be changing in the young, who know that they too will face being old and sick:

April 3, 1988   We have two dearest wishes. One is to extend our lives to meet our heart's desire, the other to live tolerably healthy lives and remain functional. We are not granted either wish wholly. One might say that aging is the price we pay for the chutzpah of remaining alive after the organism—a thing of splendor at the prime of life—starts to disintegrate and becomes a thing of squalor.

Can the winter of life also be the crown of life? Perhaps Ulyssean man will someday be the answer to that question. After a youth and prime of life spent as warrior and world wanderer, Ulysses (Odysseus) came home to Syracuse to rule his provincial domain. As Tennyson picks up the Homeric tale in his *Ulysses,* his hero felt a hunger in old age which his too placid life failed to satisfy. He had a last voyage to make:

> For my purpose holds
> to sail beyond the sunset and the baths
> of all the western stars until I die—

a task (he tells his mariners)

> not unbecoming men who strove with gods.

A strong case can be made for the "Ulyssean adult" as embodying qualities that a youth-oriented culture has shortchanged. We now emphasize the distilled wisdom of the older Odysseus, born of a life of experience, in place of the crafty younger one. His symbolic last voyage suggests a bracing fillip that the later years have given to many. It is in this sense that a society like ours, with an important role for the aging, can lay claim to "Ulyssean man" as a prime symbol.

The clue lies in the creative old, whose lives have been warrant of what is possible not only for artists, poets, thinkers, but potentially for all men and women with a creative impulse. The critics use the German term *Altersstil*—elder style—for the work of Katsushika Hokusai and Tomioka Tassai, of Michelangelo, Titian, and Rembrandt, of Goya and Cézanne, of Monet and Turner, and in our own time of Georgia O'Keefe and Louise Nevelson, of Jacques Lipschitz, of Alexander Calder and Frank Lloyd Wright in their closing years.

Not only were these painters, sculptors, and architects working at their art in those years (which was true of many artists), but they reached out to a distinct style. With Goya it was the breakthrough into the savage mood of the "black pictures," with Monet the obsessive canvasses of the waterlilies, with Turner the sea dissolving into light and color. With Nevelson the "Chapel of the Good Shepherd" in New York was the climax of a resourceful career. With Lipschitz his last three projects sought, in Hilton Kramer's words, "to attain an exalted eloquence . . . a universal statement on an epic scale." In the large, the elder style moves away from the work of the early and mid-years, sometimes into a lightness and freedom from past forms, toward greater depth, intensity, imaginativeness.

This is true as well of the poets and playwrights, from Sophocles through Goethe, to Hardy, Yeats, O'Neill. Hardy moved from his great fictions to a late poetry whose unconventional rhythm matched a craggy philosophy. In the poem "An Ancient to Ancients," he expressed his kinship with a diverse group of past writers and thinkers:

> . . . Though ours be failing frames,
>> Gentlemen,
> So were some others history names
> . . .
> Sophocles, Plato, Socrates,
>> Gentlemen,
> Pythagoras, Thucydides,
> Herodotus and Homer—yea,

> Clement, Augustine, Origen,
> Burnt brightlier toward their setting day,
> Gentlemen.

The faculty we call creativity doesn't wax with youth and maturity and wane with aging. It is *age-specific:* each age has its own kind of creativeness, for women as for men, from childhood to the end. The example of the painters and writers suggests that the creativity of the old doesn't have to be a diminished continuation of what was done better earlier. It has its own character and style, which comes from coping with the near presence of death and the preciousness of what time remains.

There are common folk—"Grandma" Moses comes most readily to mind—who started to paint, write, teach, preach, in their late decades. The closeness of the end, whatever its anxieties, may open the mind and spirit to a new sense of freedom and the use of untapped resources.

That the view from eighty-five and ninety and beyond cannot be a niggardly or fractious one was impressed on me at my sixty-fifth college reunion, at Yale, when I rose at a dinner to address my little residual band of classmates. They were in their latter eighties (I was, at eighty-five, the class youngest). I had a few notes for the talk, including some memories of social exclusion in our student years. But standing there, seeing the little cluster of my classmates who had coped with life's scarrings and braved infirmities very much like my own to get there, that segment of my talk seemed suddenly irrelevant. Aging, like combat in war, is a great simplifier and equalizer. It brings a long perspective, abbreviating the less important, leaving only life's essentials.

The trouble with reunions, as with other rituals of advancing age, is their backward-looking farewells to earlier experiences.

My instinct is not to give them much weight. Work, functioning, serenity, love, joy—these are what Jung, at eighty-five, termed "the dominants which rule human existence throughout the milleniums." I taught at Sarah Lawrence with Joseph Campbell, one of Jung's disciples, when we were both in our early thirties. Just before his death, at eighty-two, Campbell did a series of conversations with Bill Moyers which were filled with Jungian perspectives on aging, God, and death. He summed them up in a single recipe for life, "Follow your bliss."

I put Jung's "dominants" somewhat differently in a journal note:

> *January 7, 1986*   If the young dream dreams, the old see visions of what can be—but only within a reality principle they have had to learn, to their sorrow. There is a lightness of resolution in becoming old. Things that once seemed impossibly knotty somehow get resolved. It is when you have yourself been sternly tested in relation to events, family, and friends—and they in relation to you—that you are surer of them and yourself. Testing is all. . . . At this point life acquires an economy, gets stripped of the inessential. You travel light, discard your accumulated surplus anxiety and rage, get rid of the encumbering baggage of life's heavy protocols. This becomes a new personal polity, with power, rank, and status cut to the bone. You win a new freedom from labels and slogans, even from those of your own intellectual gang. . . . Thus equipped you are somewhat fitter to meet the inevitable batterings that age inflicts on the body, fitter also to respond with a mind more seasoned by adversity. You might even learn to confront Death when He comes offering to be your fellow traveler.

12. Confronting Death, Asserting Life

So here it is at last, the Distinguished Thing!

— Henry James (after his stroke)

I'm not afraid to die. I just don't want to be there when it happens.

— Woody Allen

Do not go gentle into that good night,
Old age should burn and rave at close of day,
Rage, rage against the dying of the light.

— Dylan Thomas

We live in the moment and forget the skull at the banquet.

— William James

The two great principles governing existence: what comes into being will have an end, and the mystery of this stream of being is impenetrable.

— Eric Voegelin

A T THE START OF this narrative I quote from Jacob's wrestling with the angel of God, and his emergence from that fateful night, scathed but triumphant: "For I have seen God face to face, and my life is preserved."

It is the theme of this memoir that all illness and healing, all aging, all living and dying, are a wrestling with the angel. We get wounded and are preserved—or not. But always the frame is a double one, of life and death as adversaries, but also as polar phases of each other.

Jacob's unique night and his emergence at daybreak define both frames. There have been many interpretations of the passage in the literature of Biblical criticism. My own emphasis is on Jacob's death/life testing by God in the guise of his messenger, after Jacob's own self-testing in his reconciliation with his brother Esau. But in a larger sense the shrinking from a full encounter with the angel, whether of death or life, becomes a form of death-in-life, while the recurring and pervasive denial of death becomes in the end a denial of life itself. In life-threatening crises the task is to fight death without denying its reality and the preciousness it lends to life, while at the same time asserting life.

In the cosmic drama of our lives, Death plays the heavy and dominates the stage. The curtain is never in doubt: the question is not whether it will in the end come down, with Death in possession of the stage, but how late or soon, and in what fashion. Yet we cannot, when young, make death credible to ourselves: death is real, but it is others, not we, who die.

There is an intellectual part of me which was obsessed for years with the death literature of the Greek and Elizabethan playwrights and the seventeenth-century English divines, a part which was startled by my illness into a recognition that it applied to me, too. There is another part—the sheer animal

faith—which asserts that I am not subject to these sickly cere-
brations.

A September 1986 journal entry suggests the tenacity of this
animal faith:

> Conversation at table about reaching 2000. I was of
> course the vulnerable one. Yet I declared that when I
> am feeling pretty well, like now, I find it unimaginable
> that I will die. Cognitively I know I will, with my
> logical-rational brain center, but organismically I
> cherish the unexamined faith that I am here forever.

A little more than a year later, after my eighty-fifth birthday
celebration, my daughter Joanna Townsend, in an amused, affectionate way, hit on what animated my struggle against death:
"R. asked Joany how come my continuing high spirits at my
doddering age. I like Joany's answer: 'My father can't imagine a
world without him.' " Many, if less cockily, will share this
equating of the world's existence with their individual consciousness.

But whatever the rhetoric of bravado we may thrust at death,
there is a reality of death that each of us meets in a characteristic way. We are in general a long-lived family. My grandmother
in Russia, Gita Raisse, lived to be 100 and died of shock (as the
family tradition goes) when Hitler's troops invaded her little
village. My father's death and my mother's, two years apart,
occurred in my mid-fifties, but they seemed part of the natural
order of things. Both were in their late eighties, had lived lives
of struggle and work in Russia and America, and seemed ready
for death. Coming out of a coma, my father's last words to me
were, "They are calling me from Zion." My oldest sister, Ida
Borish, clung to life with a worn-out heart until ninety-two.

Sylvia Williams, two years her junior, and just as tenacious of life, died two years later at the same age.

It was different with the death of my brother Hyman. The reality of death came hard to me as a nine year old in a wintry Catskill house, watching as my brother, three years older, gasped out his life on the sick bed next to the only stove, with the sobbing family clustered around. Hyman had developed a rheumatic heart as a boy of eight or nine, working overhard as part of an immigrant family, delivering milk at night in Bayonne. He caught pneumonia in a punishing farm winter, and his heart wasn't sturdy enough to tide him over it.

It was my primal death scene, marking the clear start of the death-line that runs through every life, consciously or not. "After the first death there is no other." As we huddled forlornly the next day around Hyman's grave, I thought I could never again have an experience to compare with it, and it has all but remained true.

The exception was my daughter Pamela, who died at twenty-nine, a young wife and mother. Like Hyman she had not learned to die. She was a sensitive, aesthetically talented girl. At college she developed a cancer of the thyroid. After intensive radiation it appeared to be contained. She married, had two children, looked forward to a promising life. But the cancer returned and spread to her lungs.

What I felt most about Pamela's death—as about Hyman's a half-century earlier—was the enormity of the blow, which matched my powerlessness to prevent it. I raged, raged, against the dying of their light. The two deaths established the pattern of my basic case against death. The injustice of these young deaths in the cutting off of potentials seemed more poignant than the snuffing out of the skills and insights accumulated by those who live longer.

That was the death-line which has stayed with me. The ways

in which we experience the death of others defines, of course, how we face our own. True, I was neither nine nor twenty-nine but just short of seventy-eight when my first cancer struck and my own death loomed. "Just when I had begun to understand the wind instruments," said Franz Joseph Haydn, wistfully. I too felt I had just found my stride. By a stark displacement I saw in my own death not the death of my parents but what I had felt in the deaths of my brother and daughter.

I now see how much I had fixed on early and unjust deaths as the very paradigm of mortality. Unlike Hamlet, death was not for me the "undiscovered country." I felt instead that it limited further discoveries in our lives, cutting them short. Historically it was the young deaths that struck my imagination—Mozart, Keats, Emily Dickinson, Randolph Bourne, John Reed, William Bolitho, Franz Kafka, John and Robert Kennedy, Martin Luther King.

They haunt me, I think, because I mourn any portion of life unreasonably and unjustly denied, which subtracts from the life as dreamt. For what we strain for in our lives is what we long for as we face death. The poet wants to write the great poem he has envisioned, the lover to make the final romantic conquest, the researcher to complete his grand research, the composer to write the ultimate symphony, the architect to build the structure of his dreams.

James Joyce tells us that "history is a nightmare from which I am trying to awake." The history of a life-menacing illness has a similar nightmare quality. For me it came with the wild contingency of the tumor, the harrowing search for its source, the torment of choices, and always the hard immediacy of Death as the Adversary to be placated, outwitted, forever to be fought— the master of the scene, preparing a reception for me. As this retrospective journal entry suggests, I was determined at least for some time to disappoint him:

I am amused at what I was supposed to feel as I faced death. The thanatologists I read tell me my first phase had to be total *terror,* followed by *denial* and *despair,* followed by *bargaining* (with doctors, fate, God), followed by some kind of *resolution,* whether in terminal rage, or surrender, or what my head nurse in intensive care at Southampton called the "Dying Swan" syndrome. . . . It is suggestive but not really a good fit for what actually happened in one mind. Yes, I had a few flashes of rage, Dylan Thomas-style, but I didn't sustain them. Rage can be cleansing, but it gets boring after a while when it turns into self-pity. I tried not to bargain or surrender, nor yet to go for that acceptance-with-dignity stuff and play the Dying Swan. . . . I tried to summon what inner resources I had in fighting not only the tumors but doubt and despair and statistical defeatism. I found an ally—when the time came—in the mind-body healing process. During the worst stretches I fought mostly by continuing to write and teach and rejoice in the gift of life. . . . To Hell with the thanatologists and their schemas! It was the only way I knew to face and outface the Adversary, Death, with whom I had to come to terms—but not (if I could help it) on his terms alone.

I add contrasting case histories of how two writers I value faced their deaths. One was Gregory Bateson, student of Balinese culture, of the behavior of dolphins and otters, of the "double-bind" in family systems—a generalist's generalist.

In an interview with Daniel Goleman, Bateson talked about his then impending death. He had rejected both chemotherapy and radiation for his cancer, because he wanted to keep his mind clear to finish a last book he was writing. Besides, on principle he was ready to die.

When his interviewer probed the reasons for his readiness, Bateson was very sure of his ground:

In the end we live by the self-limiting nature of individuals. It's very important that I shall die: you need me to. . . . If I stick around I'd go on writing books and putting words on blackboards, and, in the end, there'd be no room left for you or anyone else to put words on blackboards. . . . As they say in New Guinea, "The shit would come up to the floor." This is the moral to their myth about the origin of death. You see, the people I studied in New Guinea live on platform houses that are built eight feet off the ground. If you want to go in the middle of the night, especially if it is raining, you move a floorboard, squat over the gap, go, and go back to bed. According to the myth, people were immortal until, finally, the shit came up to the level of the floor. At this point they decided that death was necessary.

I am unpersuaded by Bateson's argument from the evolutionary necessity of self-limitation. The crowding comes from too many births, rather than from too late deaths. There is room in this society for me and for you. I don't have to stop putting words on blackboards so that you can put up a blackboard of your own. In fact, the longer we both manage to live, the greater the chance that we can learn from each other's blackboards.

There is a moving footnote to Bateson's last days. Goleman tells how two friends of Bateson met in the corridor outside his hospital room. Ram Dass believed in easing death as a spiritual passage for the terminally ill, while Kenneth Pelletier believed in the art of healing by visualizing the tumor. Bateson's wife, Lois, told Goleman that "Ram was there to help Gregory die, Ken to help him live . . . and Ken is winning."

He didn't win, nor did Ram Dass. Death won. Yet despite his

vivid New Guinea myth, I am happy that Bateson made the choice, after all, of claiming life in the face of death.

I do not equate Death with a Satanic principle of evil. I see him rather as something sacral, part of the veil of the cosmos I cannot pierce, a stern judge administering inexorable laws. Nor is he an abstraction separable from life. He is part of life's experience, the final experience.

One of the strangest greetings ever offered to death is attributed to my second writer Henry James. I quote from the account of his biographer, Leon Edel:

Early in the morning of Thursday, 2 December 1915, James' maid . . . heard the Master calling. She entered his bedroom. He was lying on the floor, his left leg had given way under him. . . . Edith Wharton reported he told (a friend) . . . that in the very act of falling he heard in the room a voice which was distinctly . . . not his own, saying "So here it is at last, the Distinguished Thing."

Who but a novelist, with a haunting sense of tradition, would have used that particular phrase after emerging from a major stroke? Yet the phrase has meaning in describing an attitude toward death that many have felt: that it is the distinctive working out of the life experience, when the quality of the life will be reflected in the style of the death. An antithesis of the Dylan Thomas "rage" against death, it is a serene acceptance of its unique finality.

There are few, seriously ill, watching for Death's possible approach, who have not at some point prepared themselves to say, "So here it is at last!" Where I differ from James is in his noun. Far from regarding Death as a "thing," I personalize him, as so many have done in dwelling on Death's meaning. Emily Dickinson left a somber portrait of Death coming for her in a horse-drawn carriage:

> Because I could not stop for Death—
> He kindly stopped for me—
> The Carriage held but just Ourselves—
> And Immortality . . .

Others have seen death arriving as a phantom rider on a phantom horse. I like the immediacy of Thomas Wolfe's "I have seen the Dark Man very close."

During my illness Death became almost a familiar: he and I drew closer together as I came to terms with my mortality. In keeping with the Jewish tradition, I veered between I–Thou talks with him and a feeling of awe for the Angel of Death, who is at times one with the Angel of God. The rabbinical legends about Old Testament heroes recount God's vow that Moses will die in the wilderness without seeing the Promised Land, and the efforts of Moses to dissuade God from carrying it out. The argument between them was long and labyrinthine. Moses used every possible trick to persuade God to repeal the sentence of his appointed death, but God was wily, and besides He had the power. Moses called on every force of Nature to intercede for him, but the intercessions were in vain. Fighting to the end, he accepted his doom only when his powers of discourse and his wisdom had been passed on to his successor, Joshua.

In a similar vein King David, seeking to learn the day of his death, was told only that he would die at seventy, on a Sabbath. Determined to outwit the Angel of Death, he postponed it week after week by busying himself every Sabbath in the study of the Torah, which gave him at least a temporary immunity from the Angel. But the Angel, insistent and cunning, contrived in the end to distract David from his studies by a noise in the garden. As David descended the palace staircase, it collapsed and he was killed.

In both instances the response to the command of the Angel

of Death was, in effect, "Don't you see how involved I am with the work of God, and how many depend on me? Go away! I'm not ready." That was, I confess, my own response when the angel came knocking. He found me, despite my illness, in the midst of life. I was neither prophet nor king, nor was I involved with the work of God, yet I was nonetheless unready to be summoned from my worldly joys and plans.

For me it was a question of incompletions. Of the books half-written: I felt their structure and shape in my very bone and wanted to see them whole. Of my children, and their children in turn: I wanted to see how the drama of life would unfold for them. Of the great world events I was watching: I wanted to see how the plot would turn out. Of the essential meaning of existence: if life is a suspense story, I wanted to read further and uncover the critical clue.

Even Moses and David, with all their worldly power and their pipeline to God, couldn't stonewall His angel indefinitely. In the end each had to open the doors wide. Immanuel Kant spoke jokingly of the "regime of reprieves" he had received from his doctors. Like Moses and David, I got several reprieves from the Angel. Like them I can't count on his continuing them indefinitely.

My father used to tell me some of these stories of the Malech h'amovits, the Angel of Death. In his opinion it was a question of being fully engaged in life. "If you run fast enough," he said, "the Angel won't be able to catch up with you." I loved my father, but I feared he was wrong.

Yet on second thought, was he? The Biblical commentators, sitting in their Yeshivas, arguing over ancient texts, were wise men. They wouldn't have composed the stories about their heroes and the Angel of Death for fun. Granted, they were saying that even lawgivers and kings, with all their power, can't bargain with Death forever. But could they have been saying more? That it is exactly when you are running fast, immersed in life, that you dare ask for a reprieve from death, to live fully a bit longer?

If the answer is even a tentative yes, it may offer a clue to the elusive mystery of the mind-body connection and its impact on the healing process. What heals us, granting us reprieves, postponing Death for a time, may be after all—as with Moses and King David—our fierce will to live.

How does a philosopher deal with death, and how does he die? In an account of illness and healing I take my examples from several figures, great and less great, in the modern tradition of therapy.

Sigmund Freud became a philosopher of death after his years as a philosopher of sexuality, which is to say that in the end he embraced the death principle to round out his embrace of Eros as the principle of desire and life. The shift, begun in *Beyond the Pleasure Principle* and completed in *Civilization and Its Discontents,* was also marked in his own life by his sense of waning powers as he coped with his cancer of the mouth and the approach of death. One might argue that Freud's later writings followed the trajectory of his illness and rationalized it. Yet the wonder is how a philosopher, like a novelist or playwright, manages to turn the dross of his own immediate experience into the metal of universals. While what came out of it was reductionist, I regard his reduction of the cosmos to the life-force and the death-drive as the kind of deepening and simplifying that sometimes comes with the late years of creative figures.

Freud raised the question of whether the purposes of life can be fulfilled without a death principle which is "pressed into the service of Eros." Both principles were "irreducible" for him, both gods "immortal," and neither could be even conceived without the other. Death is as necessary a condition for life to have purpose and meaning with its Yea as life is for death to function with its Nay.

"You've got to accentuate the positive," the popular song tells us, and "eliminate the negative." Yet the logic of saying that the second imperative must complete the first is too surfacy. Someone battling with death must strive to affirm life, but not by eliminating death as the negative. Like others, I had to confront and incorporate the illness principle into my self-healing, the death principle into my life assertion.

Among the Left-Freudian thinkers, Norman O. Brown dealt with the life/death theme, both in his *Life Against Death* and his *Love's Body,* in a way that didn't satisfy me because it was too cavalier about death. An entry from one of my reading journals may be of interest here:

I have finally dug up again Brigid Brophy's devastating critique of Norman Brown's *Love's Body,* written in 1966, and with it her dissent from the book, asserting the three things that Thanatos does for Eros: (1) "The intellectual power of asserting 'not,' of negating a proposition. Without it thought, magic and hypothesis would be impossible" (and, may I add, the No-Yes search of the computer chip). (2) The division of *self* from *not self,* on which individual personality depends. (3) "Without Thanatos there would be no Art—a specialized type of hypothesis, a figment we know to be unreal but can contemplate by grace of the label, 'fiction' . . ."

My own emphasis is not only on the "intellectual" but on the *real* power of asserting *not;* I am tempted to call Thanatos the *is not* principle. But I note that as

such it has as much *isness* as the *is so* principle. Death
asserts the *not* to us. But if we have any spirit we
assert it in turn to death. In dialectical terms it spells
the *negation of the negation.* . . . That's what I've been
doing to death, I suppose, through all these years—
negating its negation. That's what I hope to be doing
until I can do it no longer, for the one advantage death
has over life is to claim the last word. Or shall we say,
with Brando, the "Last Tango?" . . . Perhaps. Yet I
prefer the Munch painting of the dialectical dance of
life and death, with the pair of lovers in embrace, and
the new dancer entering the scene as the Dürer-like
Death figure exits.

There is in fact a dance of death as well as of life. The dance
theme runs through the great religions, notably of Dionysus in
Greece and of Siva in Hinduism. The ethnologists have found it
in every form of tribal worship, from Indonesia to the native
American tribes. Myth has it that Jesus danced on his way to
the tomb. In the Middle Ages there were depictions on the
tombs of people dancing with the dead. It got stretched ulti-
mately to a dance with one's own decaying corpse. This element, of the erotic as part of the reality of death, is true in the
history of Jewish mysticism, as it is in the life-affirming dances
of Chassidic Judaism. The swathe it cuts across religions is
evidence of how essential the mythic dance of death and of life
is to the human enterprise.

Trying to assert the *not* to death, as it does to us, and thus to
enter a dialectical dance with it, is a resolution of sorts. There is
no one particular point at which we come to terms with our
mortality. Yet when it happens—if it happens—it is a water-
shed event. Those who have been to war—and survived—have

worked it out on the battlefield. The scanty Holocaust survivors worked it out in the death camps. But for the rest, especially those with a life-threatening illness, there are few heroics in it, only a hard, continuing daily struggle.

"We receive anxiety like a Grand Hotel," wrote W. H. Auden. Part of that reception, in the early 1970s, the high point of existential *Angst,* was the recognition given to Ernest Becker's *The Denial of Death* (1973). It was a cry of affirmation to face physical and mental illness by facing and outfacing the reality of death. It got a Pulitzer, was a critical triumph, and became an American death classic. Like Gregory Bateson, Becker gave his readers a chance to test their thinking against his own, in this case in a death-bed conversation with Sam Keen which is a model of the interviewing art.

The scene is a Vancouver hospital, the time early December 1973. After some stormy years teaching the human sciences at Berkeley and San Francisco State in the later 1960s, Becker moved to a Canadian university and finished the *Denial* manu-script (his eighth book, his first big score). At the height of his success, a year later, the cancer struck. Sam Keen, an editor of *Psychology Today,* learned that Becker was dying, flew to Van-couver, and they spent "a day of loving combat" together. The entire interview is worth studying, especially since its interlocu-tors, both products of the intellectual turmoil of the 1960s, had read and thought deeply about a wide array of psychologists and philosophers on the theme of death.

The element of theater in it was that a philosopher who had thundered against the "denial of death" was now face to face with it. He had seen himself as one of the "self-realized" rather than the "everyday people." He belonged to the "obsessed" who "have to write another book . . . grow, improve."

BECKER: I mean, here is the proof of that. I am lying in a hospital bed dying and I am putting everything I have got into this interview, as though it were really important, right?

Earlier he had said that "each of us constructs a characteristic armor," and that its purpose was "to shield ourselves from the devastating awareness of our helplessness and the horror of our inevitable death." At one point Keen challenged him:

KEEN: You seem to overstress the terror of life and undervalue the appeal. Life, like sexuality, is both dreadful and desirable.
BECKER: Well, all right . . . my words have a certain iconoclastic bias. If I stress the terror it is only because I am talking to the cheerful robots. I think the world is full of too many cheerful robots who talk only about joy and the good things.

It was the first major attack the interviewer had made, and Becker's answer was a faltering one. Few of us count ourselves as "cheerful robots," yet we know there is joy in life as well as terror. Now Keen was ready for "another critical probe," as he put it.

KEEN: You say man lives on two levels: he is an animal and a symbol maker, hence he lives in one world of fact and another of illusion. . . . Symbolic knowledge is the highest form of knowledge we have. How can you justify the position that the factual world elicits only primal terror and certainty of the finality of death? The fact is, we do not know. As Kierkegaard might have said, "Where do you, Ernest Becker, a historical individual, stand in order to give so certain a separation of fact and illusion?"
BECKER: Yes, I see . . . I don't really know how to answer that. What you are saying is that the symbolic transcendence of death may be just as true as the fact of death.

It was the turning point of the dialogue. The rest was anticlimax. Becker spoke of the lack of communication between people: "It is works like Samuel Becket's *Endgame* that give a true picture of the human condition—the terrible, hopeless isolation of people."

KEEN: Your personal philosophy of life seems to be a Stoic form of heroism.

BECKER: Yes, though I would add the qualification that I believe in God.

The pathos of it was that Becker, after "dropping one book after another into the void," had finally caught the world's attention.

BECKER: . . . and now I won't be around to see these things. It is the creature who wants more experience, another ten years, another five, another four, another three. I think, gee, all these things going on and I won't be part of it.

One need not be a philosopher or therapist to move beyond the denial of death to a genuine confrontation. Many everyday people are learning to do it, learning to fight off death, yet finally to come to terms with it, to reconcile the ultimate certainty of a victory for Thanatos with the hunger for Eros, for life and more life, that even Becker acknowledges at the end.

The reader will recall the mock visualizing battles I fought out between the destroyer and preserver cells, the forces of light and darkness. I pick up from that episode in a journal note:

October 18, 1985   From this it was only a logical step to welcome the Great Intervener into the battle. It took some doing at the time. My gang had all but ousted God, saying "No anthropomorphism! You can't be foolish enough to think of God as a venerable old man with a beard. If you want to bring him back, bring him as a 'Principle' . . ." That's what I had done for some time. I had a sense of awe and reverence for a cosmos whose mystery baffles our comprehension. I even tried to think of God as an energy field. . . . But when I got sick it didn't work. It was too distant. . . .

Curiously I began bootlegging the *personal* figure of God. It was a carryover from my visualizing of the battles, and from the human imagery that haunts and infests the night—asleep, awake, and in between.

So there I was talking with God in the old Jewish pattern, from Job to Herzog, and finding him vividly an Old Testament figure indeed. It was the Buber I-Thou dialogue, but with a dash of Kierkegaardian "fear and trembling" thrown in. God knows I had *tsores* (troubles) enough to have played Job. But I didn't relish carrying on his argument with God. . . . My role was that of a respectful, affectionate subject of a King who watches over humans as well as ruling them. I started talking to Him each time I had to undergo some critical test that medical science had contrived for me. When I came through it I started thanking Him: "Thank you, dear God"—not that I had actually asked Him for anything. I figured He knew my thinking.

That was the start of the one-way conversations I have carried on since with God, broadening them into almost daily and nightly occurrences. I began to talk with Him during the wondrous brief ritual pause before I fall asleep, when I survey the day as a general might survey the field after the battle is over.

This may strike some as my form of prayer, but I didn't see it that way:

August 16, 1988   My dialogue didn't arise out of an acquisitive greed for something from the Great Giver:

"Grant me, God!" When I feel an impulse to say it I stop myself. I don't ask Him for any grants, as if He were a foundation. . . . Why then do I say "Thank you, God," in starting our conversations? My thanks during my illness were for helping me in my struggles to get through crises. My thanks still go to His caring, within reason, for me and my loved ones. I see Him as a caring God—else why would I persist in talking with Him? Omniscient? Perhaps, since I feel He knows me among the hundreds of millions. But I am not concerned with anything like His omnipotence, whether to grant or withhold. Maybe He is omnipotent, maybe He isn't. He is part of a pattern of the universe, which He may also have established. But the pattern includes my death, and alas, the deaths of many I have held dear.

It is the pattern question that most troubled me, whether there is a design in the universe, and what it is. During the early 1940s I was involved as a member of an ad hoc national committee, in an organized, sustained effort to save the Jews of the Holocaust. It failed. As a war correspondent, at forty-two, I visited Dachau, and the memory stayed with me. It was hard to believe, after that, in a benevolent design—or any design at all. When my daughter Pamela died, the genocide question, Where was God at Auschwitz?, got attenuated to a single death of cancer, yet its intensity was undiminished: it became, Where was God when Pam died?

Yet, despite my despair, the two were incommensurable. There was no principle of evil operating in the death of a young woman still on the threshold of life. But a principle of evil—radical evil—did operate at Auschwitz.

Some religions try to resolve the problem by creating a satanic Counter-God, of malevolence. Psychologists talk of the "neocortical" brain, added over time to the "primal" brain, using its destructiveness for evil purposes. Philosophers and historians focus on a distorted, false utopianism, which leads to the dystopias of human engineering, whether in Hitler's genocide or Stalin's starving and slaughter of the kulaks, or the calculated killing fields of Cambodia.

This got me somewhere, but not far enough. Instead of a benevolent God incapable of curbing evil, we had two contending Gods, of radical good and radical evil. As for man—a reflection of God—we had a man who was neither a fallen angel nor a risen ape but an amalgam of both, with both the caring and killer drives in his genes, brain, soul.

The seventeenth-century thinkers speculated about where, in the body, the soul resided. The twentieth century, the site of more massive evil than in any century of human history, came up with the figure of the "ghost in the machine." Shall we now add that there are two ghosts, and if not, then a deeply split single ghost?

If sex-in-the-head (as D. H. Lawrence called it) is a disease, then God-in-the-head may be equally so. I mean an over logical, overcognitive concept of God, rather than a simple faith in His presence. The difficulties I posed for myself in my more intellectual bouts were unresolvable. Evil in the form of man is a problem for which there is no solution, just as death is. At times I still mull over God's capacity to retain his godhead, even while failing to curb the evil in man. It was clearly of minor importance when my problem was my own illness and death, where the question of radical evil didn't enter. For a human being in trouble there is the here and now, whose claims cannot be dissolved within some grander, airier frame.

There were the dark times when I would recall A. E. Housman's bitter couplet

> And who am I to face the odds
> Of man's bedevilment—and God's?

—but it didn't make much sense to me to assign to God a deep complicity with the principle of evil, and it offered no help. That was true also of the passage in *Lear:*

> As flies to wanton boys are we to the gods,
> They mock us for their sport.

I don't say there were not moments when I felt an anger at such a cosmos. But my anger was usually directed at human agencies, including doctors, technicians, and myself—not at God, as this journal entry attests:

> *October 3, 1988* I never felt, even at the first brutal moment of "the news," that God had forsaken me. It didn't enter my head. Why should He have brought me this far, for 79 years, and suddenly dropped me into the void? I had no sense of great guilt. I didn't feel like one of the abandoned. I saw Contingency as the source of what had happened. I also knew that behind my sickness was my entire life, warts and all.

It happens with most families that they draw a circle of wagons around the sick member. I recall a phone conversation with my oldest daughter, Constance Russell. My illness startled us out of a temporary distancing which neither of us had liked. It was a healing talk:

> *October 1, 1981* A long phone conversation with Connie, calling from San Diego. She fears I will die and is aghast that it may come before we have had a chance to talk out the past between us. I am deeply moved. We had never broken off talking to each other (how could I, as her father?) but too often there has been a strain that kept us from speaking out our heart.

Now there is an authentic *cri de coeur* from her, as
never before. So we shall talk, and write each other.
. . . How many parents and children (or even friends)
are there who have adequately explained themselves
to each other before one of them dies and leaves an
aching sense of a door never opened?

The idea of breaking through the closed door of noncommunication may thus have surfaced in my mind enough for me
to raise the question about God. Thoreau's wry remark about it
is well known. Asked whether he had "made his peace with
God" his answer was: "I didn't know we had ever quarreled."
It was an evasive answer, however witty. Even without quarreling there can be noncommunication; it may even be worse than
quarreling.

For a time I used to think there was no need to talk with God
since he knew the secret and sacred sound of all things: a child's
sigh, a lover's unspoken endearments, a parent's heartbreak,
the fall of a leaf—or of a nation. Then I saw that it wasn't a very
satisfying cop-out: He might know the things I would say, but I
would miss saying them, and thereby miss out on a relation that
might define Him better for me and perhaps define me better for
Him. Herewith a journal note, written after some years of our
talk:

Are my conversations with God one-sided? Of
course—except that if God listens it is not so much *to*
me but *through* me. It would follow that he also talks
through me, even though he doesn't *to* me.

After all I don't expect Him to appear before me in a
pillar of cloud or fire. He has better things to do with
His theatrics. But my premise is that He is there because he has to be omnipresent, and that he listens,

because how else can he be omniscient? As for what he says, I have only tacit knowledge of it. . . .

If anyone were to say I am talking to myself I wouldn't dissent strongly. But since there is God in each of us I can talk with Him only by "talking to myself"—as to my *daimon*. . . . What counts is that I have reached into myself, no holds barred, and come up with griefs, failures, satisfactions, anxieties, triumphs, and shared them as with no other. . . . Having never had a therapist, I wouldn't know firsthand what one does or doesn't share with him. Anyway, God isn't my therapist. If my psyche is askew I wouldn't ask for His help in straightening me out. It would diminish Him, and keep me from distinguishing myself as a "therapeutic personality" from myself as a theological being. . . .

After these years of talking, I see God as my wiser comrade, knowing friend, shrewd and tolerant listener—however amused He must be by some of the things I bring up in our colloquies. . . . Yet with it all, His abiding mystery remains.

During my high school and college days I read the great writers of the Roman empire, and with them the classic myths. Out of it came a perverse hankering for the world of plural gods, or even of the medieval saints, with whom a mere mortal could identify more readily than with the blinding effulgence of a single God. Lacking them I was willing to settle for a world of angels, of whatever complexion, those of darkness and of light together. I held to a kinship between them, as with Rilke's plea after a spell of therapy: "If my devils are to leave me, I am afraid my angels will take flight as well."

From this pluralist theology of mine, more playful than dead earnest, one serious residue did emerge during the 1970s, before my illness. It was the *daimon* of Socrates:

> *October 7, 1983*   Talking with my *daimon*. Socrates started it, with his idea of a characteristic spirit within each of us, guiding and guarding us. A "best friend"? A "second self"? A little of each but a good deal more. . . . I have carried the idea around for a couple of decades. I talked first of it at the start of my workshops and seminars in the early 1970s. I have come to think of it finally as the part of myself that carries the message of where I am coming from, who I am, where I am going. . . . My *daimon* has been my constant companion, friend, critic, interlocutor: taunting, recklessly caustic at times, tender and caring at others. . . .

Why then do I engage in a one-sided conversation with God when I can have a pretty talky *daimon* at my command? Exactly because my *daimon* is too much myself, my twin brother. God is anything but that. "A force, not ourselves, that makes for righteousness" was how Matthew Arnold defined God. I am not sure about being righteous, but I need someone, not myself, who has at once empathy and judgment, who is detached yet receptive, who carries authority in a way my *daimon* can't. . . . As Martin Buber put it (in his "I-Thou" concept): God is the only *You* whose authority never erodes and who can never become *It.*

The presence of God for me has been the presence of a force, not myself, whom I can't kid or deceive. He is a force that has designed the universe but is also subject

to its laws, containing within His expansive self both
the Yea and Nay but at ease with His own contradic-
tion. . . . I don't "worship" Him, just as I don't pray to
Him. I live with Him and He chooses to live with me.
It is part of the prime contract of life . . . stronger and
earlier than anything in Hobbes or Rousseau, whose
"social contract" dealt with how men have to live
with each other. The *I-Thou* contract deals with how
they can live with themselves, through God in each.

I have been writing here of my feelings about God during
these last difficult years, my premise being that my illness had
everything to do with it. But how about the fact, recognized by
most witnesses to our time, that the 1970s and 1980s played host
to a worldwide wave of religious feeling that can only be called
a *return to the sacral?* Can it then have been something other
than my illness experience that shaped the change in me?

We don't do our thinking and feeling in a vacuum. I am part
of my time, subject to its influences. Yet I am also myself,
shaped by personal experience within a frame set by my society.
And my deepest personal experience during these years was my
illness:

> *October 7, 1983*   I sometimes wonder at my cheek in
> writing of God and myself in these journals. But I am
> not alone. Anyone who has been really sick knows
> that the presence of God is the realest presence of all,
> realer than doctors, nurses, procedures, realer even
> than the support of friends and intimates. . . . That is
> why I have come to call God the "great Intervener"
> for anyone sick, mediating between him and his ill-
> ness, spurring the self-healer in him.

There is another dimension of God for me, however, which flowed from His presence. It is the sense of the sacral, which invested life with a fresh wonder for me:

> *August 26, 1988*   For some time after my journeyman days with Machiavelli and the power thinkers I began to see the other pole of power—the transcendent source of life from which it sprang. But when you learn transcendence not in the books but in the experience of a fight for life, it takes on a different meaning. . . .
>
> My illness gave the idea of the sacral in my life a depth it lacked in the classroom. One might agree with Durkheim that "the contrast between sacred and profane is the widest and deepest the human mind can make." Yet for myself I find all sorts of things now— even "profane" things—to be sacred. Our few acres of grass and trees at White Hedges, whether morning, dusk or full moon—I get a shiver of delight from gazing at them. I expand it to the larger plot of land I call my country, with its own brand of sacredness. I look at the old sundial on the lawn, and know it is always later than I think, and the dial becomes an image of the sacredness of time itself, of which so little remains. The sacral is the ritualizing of all the things—small and large—that are invested with life's essential meaning. . . . If I had to sum up in a phrase the difference my illness made in me, it would be that I have become the familiar of the sacral, and that every day of my life has learned to carry its own transcendence.

I turn back now to the days after my heart attack. The scene is the hospital at Southampton, the time July 4, 1984. I had entered it with a middle-of-the-night infarction (see Chapter 9). At dawn the next morning my son Steve caught the "milk train" from New York, checked the hospital arrangements, and called my wife Jenny in London to tell her things were under control. That day Michael arrived from Virginia, where he had been conducting a cancer retreat, and the next day they showed up together in my cubbyhole room at intensive care.

I had not quite expected the conversation that followed, which I reconstructed as faithfully as I could:

> Michael and Steve today, my oldest and next-born sons, manly, loving. . . . Michael began: "Dad, would you mind if we talk about the immortality of the soul?" I was amused, intrigued. Michael continued: "You're as tough a nut for death to crack as we've always thought. Do you believe that when you die, whatever happens to your physical body, your soul will live on?"

I savored the moment. Here was a conversation on immortality in a hospital setting of living and dying.

> I asked Michael what his belief was. "I come at it out of the Yoga tradition," he said. "I am not certain of the soul's immortality. What I am certain of is that my soul is central to who I am. I see it as the observing, energetic place, free of immediate personal memories and daily concerns. . . . It is a place from which many, in the course of history, have observed life. This observer within us can be replaced—rebuilt —in many energetic patterns that I cannot know now. I do know that the self that looks through me on the world has looked on the world through many others before me, as an observing pattern of energy. That's

why I feel that the place from which I now see the world is one from which I will see the world again and again." . . . I had heard fragments of this from him before but never as fully.

I asked Steve, knowing he would have his own view; and he did: "I don't think death is the end. There is something beyond it," Steve said. He took the Buddhist line—"We think too much of the individual self and the individual soul in Western thought." When I pushed him it came down to "an energy field—call it the World Soul or the 'oversoul' " . . . And when he dies? "Physically I'll biodegrade," he said, true environmentalist that he was. "My soul will simply become part of the sum total of the energy field that it and I came from."

It was my turn. Here we were, two sturdy young men and their battered old father, all three of us scared about me, none admitting it. Here were my sons asking me the eschatology questions about first and last things.

I now believe I have a soul, I said, just as I believe in the reality of God in some personal form. Right now my soul and body, my brain, mind, and spirit, are functioning together, forming my total self. When I die the self dies, and all of them will cease, the soul no exception. I wished I could believe otherwise. It would be consoling to have a nice little soul around to keep me company.

Was there no way I thought I might outlive death? They pressed hard.

By metaphor, yes, I said. In how my family and friends and students remember me. Perhaps a youngster will come upon a book of mine and his blood and brain will quicken, as mine used to do—and still does—when I pick up a book with some fire in it. I quoted Samuel Butler—"Where dead men meet, on lips of living men."

It's only a metaphor, and it's not more than a wisp of immortality. But I still reach out and try to clutch it, in every class, in every piece of work I write.

Beyond the metaphor, I recall telling my sons, there was the triumph of the seed, that I would live on biologically in them, in all my daughters and sons and in theirs. The knowledge that for a few generations some traces of my memory will be passed on, from children to children, is all the certainty I want and need.

In his work on Henry James, Leon Edel has written of the "secret life myth," an intimation of the deepest self which we may rarely reveal but which guides us through our most difficult life passages. I suspect that each of us has also a secret death myth, of how we should like best to die. A journal note suggests how I have felt about this:

> How do I want to die? Not in a hospital bed. I have seen too many of them. Not even in our big Jamaican four-poster, at Southampton. I want to go, if we can manage it, at the fireplace with logs crackling, amidst talk of adventures and events in our lives. . . . Maybe some of our offspring will raise a toast, and recall common memories and family rituals.

I had written an earlier journal note about the corollary question—how I wanted to be remembered:

> I have always thought I wanted an Irish wake. . . . I remember, years ago, reading a passage in an English novel of the 1950s, whose hero wanted his friends to

gather after his death, to remember him with drink-
ing, storytelling, lovemaking. It was death celebrating
life. I haven't been able to shake it.

Several years later I picked up the thread about being remembered:

September 25, 1988   Yes, I want the *Yisgadal v'yis-
gadash shema rabbo* intoned, ritual fashion, as it was
at my father's death. It is a great sound to die by. . . .
Yet I don't want a solemn, tear-filled service, or a
memorial gathering to which people feel obligated to
come, and a few offer eulogies from notes they have
labored over. I would prefer some friends and family
to gather under the pear tree where both Steve and
Adam were married, and where my children and their
children have gathered. Perhaps someone will read
from stuff I have written, saying I lived for words.
I shall die with some pleasure at leaving words behind, along with children and their children to recall
them. When it's over, perhaps the young will go inside
and dance the dance of love and life.

NOTES

1. Contingency Is King

22   *a book on the Kennedys: Ted and the Kennedy Legend: A Study in Character and Destiny* (St. Martin, 1980).

2. The Locus of the Evil

29   *a bleak, adversarial book:* Ivan Illich, *Medical Nemesis: The Expropriation of Health* (Pantheon, 1976).

32   *The eternal ones of the dream:* The phrase is from the title of a book by Geza Roheim, a psychoanalyst and anthropologist, one of Freud's original group of disciples.

34   *Machiavelli gave the name* Fortuna: The reference is to Niccolo Machiavelli's use of the concept of Fortune, in *The Prince* and in the *History of Florence.* Machiavelli felt that the element of sheer chance in human affairs could be combated, if not overcome, by *virtù*—strength and clarity of purpose—in the leader and the state. I wrote about him in my introductory essay to the Modern Library edition of *The Prince and the Discourses* (1940).

35   *the respective paradigms we had:* I use "paradigm" in the sense Thomas

PAGE

S. Kuhn employs in *The Structure of Scientific Revolutions* (2d ed., University of Chicago, 1970), as the accepted model in our minds, and the cluster of assumptions with which we approach a problem.

3. The Torment of Choice

44 *hence my torment of choice:* I am writing here of my inner debate in 1981. If my illness had come toward the end of the decade I would have had the benefit of several books that have dealt wisely with the question of "choice in cancer." I refer to them, among others, in my *Further Reading.*

4. The Universe of the Ill

53 *I thought of Franklin Roosevelt:* It is now recognized that FDR's coping with his polio shaped much of the character and style with which he met his challenges as Governor and President. The best discussions are in Kenneth S. Davis, *FDR: The Beckoning of Destiny 1882–1928* (Putnam, 1972), and Geoffrey Ward, *A First-Class Temperament: The Emergence of Franklin D. Roosevelt* (Harper & Row, 1989).

53 *I thought also of Milton Erickson:* The greatest medical hypnotherapist, Milton H. Erickson, lived in Phoenix, Arizona, during the latter part of his life and carried on much of his work in a wheelchair. See Jay Haley, *Uncommon Therapy: The Psychiatric Technique of Milton H. Erickson, M.D.* (Norton, 1986).

5. Don't Take My Night Away

62 *important research in . . . psycho-neuro-immunology:* These were earlier scientific papers in the field through the 1970s, as reprinted in S. Locke, ed., *Foundations of Psychoneuroimmunology* (Aldine, 1985). But it was not taken seriously until the 1980s.

70 *a creature who denies his creatureliness":* From Ernest Becker, *The Denial of Death* (Free Press, 1972). For a further discussion of Becker's thinking, as expressed in an interview with Sam Keen, see chap. 13, pp. 180–82.

75 *both my tumors:* For my second tumor see Chap. 6, p. 77–94.

7. "Don't Let Them Do an Abelard on You"

100 *a conference . . . on the ethics of the media:* The proceedings were published in *The Responsibilities of Journalism,* edited by Robert Schmuhl (University of Notre Dame Press, 1984).

108 *William Harvey expressed his sense of wonder:* I use Harvey's apostrophe to the heart as one of the epigraphs for Chapter 9, p. 177.

108 *We make a god of neither:* There is a sense, however, in which the champions of the immune system's glories see themselves in a Promethean role—Prometheus who rebelled against the reigning divinities and stole fire from Heaven.

109 *the masterly work of Milton Erickson in . . . "altered states":* For a discussion of this whole area of altered states, see Ernest L. Rossi, *The Psychobiology of Mind-Body Healing* (Norton, 1986). Rossi presents Milton Erickson's approach, insights from Carl Jung and dashes of "behavioral medicine" research in a challenging provisional synthesis.

110 *is found in some form in almost every culture:* See Aldous Huxley's classic anthology, *The Perennial Philosophy* (Harper, 1970). See also an insert on "The Perennial Philosophy of Healing," part of a longer piece, "The Tradecraft of Commonweal Cancer," by Michael Lerner, in *Advances* vol. 4, (1987).

8. A Medical Miracle—and a Medical Museum

115 *hanging on the hope that the process . . . will continue to be effective:* Several years ago I learned that the LHRH analog does not wholly lack dangers. In follow-up long-term research on rats (so Vincent Hollander told me) some cases of cancer had been discovered, including brain cancer. I signed the requested release, expressing a fervent wish that future rats would stay clear of all cancers.

9. "Thank God, It's Only a Heart Attack!"

129 *several talks with Dr. Dean Ornish:* Dr. Ornish's undertaking has been ambitious—to establish whether "comprehensive life-style changes can reverse coronary atherosclerosis." His answer is on the side of reversibility—that patients with coronary artery disease who follow a strict

vegetarian diet, exercise, stress reduction and group therapy show "statistically significant improvement." (See also my reference to Dr. Ornish's "reversibility" thesis on p. 138.) A book reporting on the results of his controlled study is in press. I found an earlier book of his useful—*Stress, Diet and Your Heart* (New American Library, 1982)—although I fear I did not follow his nutritional injunctions seriously enough.

129   *I read Norman Cousins'* The Healing Heart: Of Cousins' books this was the one most relevant for me after my own infarction (*The Healing Heart: Antidotes to Panic and Helplessness,* Norton, 1983). I was taken by his experience in disciplined walking, which I later put to good use for myself. I also found the four Afterwords by as many physicians a striking addition, especially the one by Dr. David S. Cannom, to whom I turned several times for help during my stays in Los Angeles.

136   *I go with James Joyce:* I refer of course to Joyce's *Ulysses,* and to Stephen Daedalus. I have been greatly influenced, in my thinking about innovativeness in healing, by the risk-taking Daedalean imagination wherever it has cropped up in recent medical advances. This applies also to my reflections on my own aging experiences and the bearing of "Ulyssean man" upon them (See Chapter 11, especially p. 163.)

10. The Upward Spiral: The Doctor Within the Patient

139   *This* shaman effect: One of the early—and still important—books on shamanism goes well beyond the sense in which I use it here. In *Shamanism: Archaic Techniques of Ecstasy* (Princeton University Press, 1964), Mircea Eliade stresses the experiences, akin to death and resurrection, that enable the shaman "to communicate his strength" to others. He was seeking—as he wrote in his journal much later (*No Souvenirs,* University of Chicago, 1977)—"to unveil the primordial world in which creations and inventions (techniques, the arts) were not yet detached from their religious matrix." It suggests some perspectives about a technological age in which the religious matrix is present only in exceptional doctors and patients. In that sense the meaningful movement of our time involves an effort to restore it more widely in both.

144   *what he lived and argued for:* The "exceptional patients" whose "self-healing" Dr. Bernie S. Siegel describes in his eloquent and vastly popular *Love, Medicine and Miracles* (Harper, 1988) doubtless saw in him

the shaman-in-the-doctor but also contained a self-regarding doctor-as-healer in themselves. Both with respect to doctor and patients it is strikingly close—although on a more sophisticated level—to the Schweitzer experience at Lambarene.

144 *"still invested with the* mysterium tremendum": The terrifying mystery. I take the phrase from Rudolf Otto's *Idea of the Holy* (Oxford, 1971). The book was published in the original German in 1917, in the midst of World War I. A considerable school of theology has developed from it, reaching to Paul Tillich, whom Otto's thinking greatly influenced.

11. Aging: The Last Voyage

146 *"That is no country for old men":* The start of William Butler Yeats' "Sailing to Byzantium," an excerpt from which is one of the epigraphs of this chapter.

148 *Robin Lehman . . . a film he was shooting":* Forever Young, a documentary by Robin Lehman, has been shown from time to time. The curious reader is directed to Opus Films, Ltd.

150 *at Bolinas . . . during one of the cancer retreats:* Our visit was to Commonweal, the ongoing holistic research and treatment project at Bolinas, California. For a description of its work, see Michael Lerner, "The Tradecraft of Commonweal Cancer," *Advances* Vol. 4, no. (1987). See also the same author's *The Geography of Hope: Maps of Choice in Cancer* (forthcoming, HarperCollins).

152 *"an aging revolution is taking place":* See *America as a Civilization, 30th Anniversary Edition, with an added chapter on "The New America, 1957–1987"* (Holt, 1987). For the section, in the original edition, on "The Middle and End of the Journey," see pp. 611–20. For the discussion in the added chapter, see "The Pursuit of Selfhood and Belief," pp. 985–1001, esp. pp. 995–97.

152 *I wrote my own responding credo:* The excerpt is from a commentary of mine on Skinner's lecture to the American Psychological Association, "Intellectual Self-Management in Old Age," *New York Post,* September 1, 1982, "Sorry, Skinner—It's All in Your Mind."

155 *a different clue in Gerald Heard:* See Gerald Heard, *The Five Ages of Man: The Psychology of Human History* (Julian Press, 1963). The chapter on "The Ordeal of Second Maturity" is of special interest.

PAGE

155 *a reprise of their famous original model:* A list of Erik Erikson's books appears in the Bibliography. For an influential insight into the aging phase of the life journey, as affected by reminiscence, see Robert N. Butler's "The Life Review: An Interpretation of Reminiscence in the Aged," *Psychiatry* 26 (February 1963): 65–76, which has generated considerable commentary. (See Kathleen Woodward, "Reminiscence and the Life Review," in Thomas R. Cole and Sally Gadow, eds., *What Does It Mean To Grow Old?* (Duke, 1986), pp. 135–61.

161 *Daniel Levinson calls his version:* See Daniel Levinson et al., *The Seasons of a Man's Life* (Knopf, 1978), especially Chapter 1, "The Life Cycle and Its Seasons," on the methodology of his approach. A companion volume, on the seasons of a woman's life, has been long in preparation.

161 *Oswald Spengler wrote:* The reference is to Spengler's *The Decline of the West,* English edition in two volumes (Knopf, 1926, 1928), one-volume edition (Knopf, 1930). The most accessible work on him for the general reader is H. Stuart Hughes, *Oswald Spengler: A Critical Estimate* (Scribner, 1952). See also a one-volume edition of the *Decline,* abbreviated, with an introductory essay by Hughes (Oxford, 1990).

161 *So careless of the single life:* The lines are from Alfred, Lord Tennyson's "In Memoriam," written at the height of the conflict between evolution and traditional religion.

162 *Robert Nisbet argues:* The reference is to his *Prejudices: A Philosophical Dictionary* (Harvard, 1983).

163 *the German term* Altersstil: I have profited here from the assessments of individual artists in Hugo Munsterberg's *The Crown of Life: Artistic Creativity in Old Age* (Harcourt Brace Jovanovich, 1983).

164 *Hardy moved . . . to a late poetry:* for Thomas Hardy's "An Ancient to Ancients," see *The Complete Poems* (Macmillan, 1982).

166 *Campbell did a series of conversations:* See Joseph Campbell, with Bill Moyers, *The Power of Myth* (Doubleday, 1988).

12. Confronting Death, Asserting Life

168 *At the start:* see the front matter for this book. I repeat it here for the convenience of the reader: "And Jacob was left alone, and there wrestled a man with him until the breaking of the day. And when he saw that he prevailed not against him, he touched the bottom of his thigh;

and the hollow of Jacob's thigh was out of joint as he wrestled with him . . . and Jacob called . . . the place Peniel, 'for I have seen God face to face, (the face of God), and my life is preserved.' " For the classic post-Biblical commentary, see Louis Ginzberg, *The Legends of the Jews*, vol. 1 chap. 6, (Jewish Publication Society, Philadelphia, 1956, "Jacob"). The reader may also find nourishment, as I did, in the classic fictional treatment of the Jacob saga, Thomas Mann's sequence of novels forming *Joseph and His Brothers* (Knopf, 1948).

170   *After the first death:* The start of a Dylan Thomas poem.

172   *In an interview . . . Bateson talked:* In *Psychology Today* (August 1978).

174   *One of the strangest greetings:* This excerpt is from Leon Edel's one-volume abridgement of his multivolumed account of James' life and art, *Henry James, A Life* (Harper, 1985), p. 706.

175   *The rabbinical legends . . . recount:* See Louis Ginzberg, *The Legends of the Jews.* Volume 3 is devoted entirely to "Moses in the Wilderness." The David legends are in volume 4.

176   *My father used to tell me:* I wrote of my father's death in a piece in *The Unfinished Country* (Simon and Schuster, 1959), pp. 7–9, "My Father Moved."

177   *as he coped with his cancer of the mouth:* The best account of Freud's illness and death are in the book by his doctor, Max Schur, *Freud: Living and Dying* (International Universities, 1972). See also Peter Gay's *Freud: A Life for Our Time* (Norton, 1988). While Freud discussed the death principle in *Civilization and Its Discontents,* he fails curiously to mention the Greek Thanatos as the polar equivalent of Eros—perhaps because Wilhelm Stekel used it extensively in Freud's circle, and Freud had broken with him.

180   *a day of loving combat:* The interview with Ernest Becker, by Sam Keen, is in *Psychology Today* (April 1974): 71–80.

183   *So there I was, talking with God:* The reference to "Herzog" is to Saul Bellow's novel by that name. For the "Buber I-Thou dialogue," see Walter Kaufman's *Martin Buber's I and Thou,* and also his *Discovering the Mind,* vol. 2, on Nietzsche, Heidegger and Buber, (McGraw-Hill, 1980), pp. 239–80.

184   *a member of an ad hoc national committee:* For the early effort to save Europe's Jews from their mass death, see an account by one of the participants, Yitshaq Ben-Ami, *Years of Wrath, Days of Glory: Memoir*

from the Irgun (1982) and his *Postscript* in a "second expanded edition" (Shengold, 1983). See also David S. Wyman, *The Abandonment of the Jews* (Pantheon, 1986). My involvement in this effort, along with my later visit to Dachau, strongly colored my perception of death.

185   *a deeply split single ghost:* I was thinking of Arthur Koestler's *The Ghost in the Machine* (Macmillan, 1967), on the urge in man to self-destruction. For a reader like myself, whose ailments had enmeshed him in pharmacological and other interventions, Koestler's final proposed remedy had a certain piquancy. It is "for salvation synthesized in the laboratory," in the form of a pill to heal the split between man's later and earlier brains, out of which (as Koestler saw it) his self-destructiveness comes. He admits that it "may seem materialistic, crankish, or naive," but adds, "there is a Jungian twist in it . . . the ancient alchemist's dream to concoct the *elixir vitae.*"

189   *From this pluralist theology:* I was aware, when I wrote this journal note and the others, of the inconsistencies they offer. I was saying that God is many, but He is also one, that God is within me, but He is also a "force, not myself, that makes for righteousness." I knew, from my reflections on the Holocaust, that the comforting feeling of a God within each of us can lead to limitless destructiveness. I knew also, from my father's discourses on the Torah, that God is a figure to evoke awe and reverence. But knowing this I knew also that God's polarities could not be contained within a single formula. From my experience with illness it was the sense of his multiform presence that counted for me.

189   *God is the only* You: For this way of putting it, see Walter Kaufmann's essay on Buber in *Discovering the Mind.*

190   return to the sacral: I have dealt more fully with this wave of religious feeling in the Afterword of *America as a Civilization* (Holt, 1987), pp. 998–1001.

191   *my journeyman days with Machiavelli:* The reference is to the Introductory Essay of my edition of Machiavelli's *The Prince and the Discourses* (Modern Library, 1940; rev. ed. 1950). It represents the "hard" side of my political thinking.

191   *"I find . . . even 'profane' things—to be sacred":* This again was part of the polar thinking that came out of my illness. For an anthropological view by a historian of religions, see Mircea Eliade, *The Sacred and the Profane* (German ed., 1957; English trans., 1959). Even in his journals, especially *No Souvenirs, 1957–1969* (Harper, 1977) and *Journal III,*

PAGE

1970–1978 (University of Chicago, 1989), Eliade is almost obsessed with his idea of the "camouflaging of the sacred in the profane": "Indeed the religious experience consists of 'tearing off the veil' and of ripping off the mask." (*Journal III,* pp. 135–36).

194   *"I quoted Samuel Butler":* From his poem, "Life After Death," which speaks of meeting "those among the dead whose pupils we have been." The last two lines: "Yet meet we shall, and part, and meet again, / Where dead men meet, on lips of living men."

194   *an English novel of the 1950s:* David Garnett, *Aspects of Love* (Aurum Press Ltd., 1955).

FURTHER READING

OVERVIEW

Achterberg, Jeanne. *Imagery in Healing.* New Science Library, 1985.

Arendt, Hannah. *The Human Condition.* University of Chicago, 1958.

Balint, Michael. *The Doctor, His Patient and the Illness.* Rev. ed. International Universities, 1972.

Barsky, Arthur J. *Worried Sick.* Little, Brown, 1988.

Borysenko, Joan. *Minding the Body, Mending the Mind.* Bantam, 1987.

Brody, H. *Placebo and the Philosophy of Medicine.* University of Chicago, 1980.

Callahan, Daniel. *Health and the Good Society.* Simon and Schuster, 1990.

———. *What Kind of Life: The Limits of Medical Progress.* Simon and Schuster, 1989.

Caplan, A. L., H. T. Engelhardt and J. J. McCartney. *Concepts of Health and Disease: Interdisciplinary Perspectives.* Addison-Wesley, 1981.

Capra, Fritjof. *The Turning Point: Science, Society and the Rising Culture.* Bantam, 1982.

———. *Uncommon Wisdom: Conversations with Remarkable People.* Bantam, 1989.

Carlson, Rick J. *The End of Medicine.* Wiley, 1975.

Cassell, E. J. *The Healer's Art.* Anchor, 1980.

Cousins, Norman. *Head First: The Biology of Hope.* Dutton, 1989.

Dossey, Larry. *Recovering the Soul: A Scientific and Spiritual Search.* Bantam, 1969.

———. *Space, Time and Medicine.* Shambala, 1983.

Dubos, René. *The Mirage of Health: Utopias, Progress and Biological Change.* Harper, 1959.

Eckstein, Gustave. *The Body Has a Head.* Harper, 1970.

Eisenberg, D. *Encounters with Qi: Exploring Chinese Medicine.* Norton, 1985.

Eliade, Mircea. *Shamanism: Archaic Techniques of Ecstasy.* Princeton, 1964.

Entralgo, P. L., L. J. Ratner and J. M. Sharp, eds. *The Therapy of the Word in Classical Antiquity.* Yale, 1970.

Ferguson, Marilyn. *The Aquarian Conspiracy: Personal and Social Transformation in the 1980's.* St. Martin, 1980.

Fess, Laurence, and Kenneth Rothenberg. *The Second Medical Revolution: From Biomedicine to Infomedicine.* New Science Library, 1987.

Foucault, Michel. *Birth of the Clinic: An Archaelogy of Medical Perception.* Pantheon, 1973.

Frank, Jerome D. *Persuasion and Healing.* Schocken, 1970.

Frankl, Victor E. *The Doctor and the Soul.* Vintage, 1965.

Fuchs, Victor R. *Who Shall Live?* Basic, 1974.

Goldstein, Kurt. *Human Nature in the Light of Psychopathology.* Schocken, 1963.

———. *The Organism.* American Book, 1939.

Haley, J., ed. *Advanced Techniques of Hypnosis and Therapy: Selected Papers of Milton H. Erickson.* Grune & Stratton, 1967.

———. *Uncommon Therapy: The Psychiatric Techniques of Milton H. Erickson, M.D.* Norton, 1986.

Hampden-Turner, Charles. *Maps of the Mind.* Macmillan, 1982.

Huxley, Aldous. *Perennial Philosophy.* Harper, 1970.

Illich, Ivan. *Medical Nemesis: The Expropriation of Health.* Pantheon, 1976.

James, William. *Varieties of Religious Experience.* Macmillan, 1961.

Jung, Carl. *Answer to Job.* Meridian, 1964.

———. *Modern Man in Search of a Soul.* Harcourt, 1933.

Kaptchuk, T. *The Web That Has No Weaver: Understanding Chinese Medicine.* Congdon & Weed, 1983.

Katz, J. *The Silent World of Doctor and Patient.* Free Press, 1984.

Knowles, John W., ed. *Doing Better and Feeling Worse: Health in the U.S.* Norton, 1977.

Koestler, Arthur. *The Ghost in the Machine.* Macmillan, 1967.

———. *Janus: A Summing Up.* Pan, 1979.

Kuhn, Thomas S. *The Structure of Scientific Revolutions.* Rev. ed. University of Chicago, 1970.

Locke, S., and M. Hornig-Rohan, eds. *Mind and Immunity: Behavioral Immunology (1976–1982).* Institute for the Advancement of Health, 1983.

Locke, S., et al., eds. *Foundations of Psychoneuroimmunology.* Aldine, 1985.

May, William F. *The Physician's Covenant: Images of the Healer in Medical Ethics.* Westminster, 1983.

Miller, Neal E. "Biomedical Foundations for Biofeedback." In John V. Basmajian, ed., *Biofeedback: Principles and Practice for Clinicians.* Williams & Wilkins, 1989.

Northrop, F. S. *The Meeting of East and West: An Inquiry Concerning World Understanding.* Oxbow, 1979.

Ornstein, Robert, and David Sobel. *The Healing Brain.* Simon and Schuster, 1987.

————. *Holiday Pleasures.* Addison-Wesley, 1989.

Pelletier, Kenneth R. *Mind as Healer, Mind as Slayer.* Delta, 1977.

Payer, Lynn. *Medicine and Culture.* Holt, 1988.

Remen, R. Naomi. *The Human Patient.* Anchor 1980.

Rodgers, David E., and Eric J. Cassell, eds. "America's Doctors, Medical Science, Medical Care." *Daedalus* (Spring 1986).

Rossi, Ernest L. *The Psychobiology of Mind-Body Healing.* Norton, 1986.

Rossi, Ernest L., and David B. Cheek. *Mind-Body Therapy: Methods of Ideodynamic Healing in Hypnosis.* Norton, 1988.

Sagan, Leonard A. *The Health of Nations.* Basic, 1987.

Salmon, J. W. *Alternative Medicines: Popular and Policy Perspectives.* Tavistock, 1984.

Selye, Hans. *The Stress of Life.* Rev. ed. McGraw-Hill, 1978.

Shaw, George Bernard. *The Doctor's Dilemma: A Tragedy.* Garland, 1981.

Shorter, Edward. *Bedside Manners: The Troubled History of Doctors and Patients.* Simon and Schuster, 1985.

Siegel, Bernie S. *Love, Medicine and Miracles.* Harper, 1986.

Simonton, Carl, et al. *Getting Well Again.* Tarcher, 1978.

Smuts, J. *Holism and Evolution.* Greenwood, 1973.

Sobel, David S. *Ways of Health: Holistic Approaches to Ancient and Contemporary Medicine.* Harcourt, 1979.

Spiro, Howard M. *Doctors, Patients, and Placebos.* Yale, 1986.

Starr, Paul. *The Social Transformation of American Medicine.* Basic, 1984.

Steeler, Miriam, and Humphrey Osmond. *Models of Madness, Models of Medicine.* Macmillan, 1974.

Taylor, Shelley E. *Positive Illusions: Creative Self-Discipline and the Healing Mind.* Basic, 1989.

Von Bertalanffy, Ludwig. *General System Theory.* Rev. ed. Braziller, 1969.

Weil, Andrew. *Health and Healing: Understanding Conventional and Alternative Medicine.* Houghton Mifflin, 1983.

Zahourek, Rothlyn P., ed. *Relaxation and Imagery: Tools for Therapeutic Communication and Intervention.* Saunders, 1988.

ILLNESS NARRATIVES, DOCTORS' NARRATIVES

Barrett, Marvin. *Spare Days.* Arbor, 1988.

Brody, Howard. *Stories of Sickness.* Yale, 1988.

Cousins, Norman. *Anatomy of an Illness, as Perceived by the Patient.* Norton, 1979.

———. *The Healing Heart: Antidotes to Panic and Helplessness.* Norton, 1983.

Hilfiker, D. *Healing the Wounds: A Physician Looks at His Work.* Penguin, 1987.

Kemenetz, Rodger. *Terra Infirma.* University of Arkansas, 1985.

Kleinman, Arthur. *The Illness Narratives: Suffering, Healing and the Human Condition.* Basic, 1988.

Konner, Melvin. *Becoming a Doctor: A Journey of Initiation in Medical School.* Viking, 1987.

Lipore, Michael J. *Death of the Clinician: Requiem or Reveille?* Charles C. Thomas, 1982.

Schreiber, LeAnne. *Midstream.* Viking, 1990.

Schur, Max. *Freud: Living and Dying.* International Universities, 1972.

Sontag, Susan. *Illness as Metaphor.* Farrar, Straus & Giroux, 1978.

Thomas, Lewis. *The Youngest Science: Notes of a Medicine Watcher.* Viking, 1983.

Tsongas, Paul. *Heading Home.* Knopf, 1984.

White, Paul Dudley. *My Life in Medicine.* Gambit, 1971.

SYMBOLIC DISEASES: METAPHORS, TREATMENT, TRANSCENDENCE

Bateson, Mary Catherine. *Thinking AIDS.* Addison-Wesley, 1989.

Benjamin, Harold J. *From Victim to Victor: The Wellness Community Guide to Fighting for Recovery for Cancer Patients and Their Families.* Tarcher, 1987.

Camus, Albert. *The Plague.* Random House, 1947.

Goffman, Erving. *Stigma, Notes on the Management of Spoiled Identity.* Simon and Schuster, 1986.

LeShan, Lawrence. *Cancer as a Turning Point: A Handbook for People with Cancer, Their Families, and Health Professionals.* Dutton, 1989.

Moore, Thomas J. *Heart Failure: A Critical Inquiry Into American Medicine and the Revolution in Heart Care.* Random House, 1989.

Ornish, Dean. *Stress, Diet and Your Heart.* New American Library, 1982.

Shilts, Randy. *And the Band Played On: Politics, People, and the AIDS Epidemic.* St. Martin, 1987.

AGING, THE LIFE COURSE, DEATH

Achenbaum, W. Andrew. *Shades of Gray.* Little, Brown, 1985.

Ariès, Philippe. *Western Attitudes Toward Death: From the Middle Ages to the Present.* Johns Hopkins, 1974.

Balter, Paul, and David Brim, eds. *Life Span Development and Behavior.* Academic, 1980.

Beauvoir, Simone de. *The Coming of Age.* Putnam, 1972.

Becker, Ernest. *The Denial of Death.* Free Press, 1973.

Bianchi, Eugene C. *Aging as Spiritual Journey.* Crossroads, 1982.

Blythe, Ronald. *The View in Winter: Reflections on Old Age.* Harcourt, 1979.

Butler, Robert N. "The Life Review: An Interpretation of Reminiscence in the Aged." *Psychiatry* 26 (February 1963): 65–76.

―――. *Why Survive?* Harper, 1985.

Callahan, Daniel. *Setting Limits: Medical Goals in an Aging Society.* Simon and Schuster, 1987.

Choron, Jacques. *Death and Western Thought.* Collier, 1963.

Clark, Kenneth. *The Artist Grows Old.* Cambridge, 1972.

Cole, Thomas R., and Sally Gadow, eds. *What Does It Mean To Grow Old: Reflections from the Humanities.* Duke, 1986.

Comfort, Alex. *The Biology of Senescence.* 3rd ed. Elsevier, 1979.

―――. *A Good Age.* Simon and Schuster Fireside, 1976.

―――. *The Process of Aging.* New American Library, 1961.

Cowley, Malcolm. *The View from Eighty.* Viking, 1980.

Erikson, Erik. *Identity and the Life Cycle.* Norton, 1980.

―――. *Identity: Youth and Crisis.* Norton, 1968.

―――. *Insight and Responsibility.* Norton, 1964.

―――. *The Life Cycle Completed: A Review.* Norton, 1982.

―――. *Life History and the Historical Moment.* Norton, 1975.

Erikson, Erik, ed. *Adulthood.* Norton, 1978.

Erikson, Erik, Joan Erikson and Helen Kivnick. *Vital Involvement in Old Age.* Norton, 1986.

Estes, Carol Lynn. *The Aging Enterprise.* Jossey-Bass, 1979.

Fingarette, Herbert. *The Self in Transformation.* Harper, 1977.

Fischer, David Hackett. *Growing Old in America.* Oxford, 1978.

Fries, James M. *Aging Well: The Life Plan for Health and Vitality in Your Later Years.* Addison-Wesley, 1989.

Gordon, Michael. *Old Enough To Feel Better: A Medical Guide for Seniors.* Johns Hopkins, 1989.

Grene, David. *Reality and the Heroic Pattern: Last Plays of Ibsen, Shake-*

speare and Sophocles. University of Chicago, 1967.

Haber, Carole. *Beyond 65: The Dilemma of Old Age in America's Past.* Cambridge, 1983.

Hall, G. Stanley. *Senescence.* Appleton, 1922.

Jung, Carl. "The Stages of Life." In *Modern Man in Search of a Soul.* Harcourt, 1933.

Keith-Ross, Jennie. *Old People, New Lives.* University of Chicago, 1977.

Kermode, Frank. *The Sense of an Ending.* Oxford, 1967.

Koenke, E. D., ed. *The Meaning of Life.* Oxford, 1981.

Kubler-Ross, D. *On Death and Dying.* Macmillan, 1969.

Levine, S. *Who Dies?: An Investigation of Conscious Living and Conscious Dying.* Anchor, 1982.

Levinson, Daniel. *The Seasons of a Man's Life.* Knopf, 1978.

Lifton, Robert. *The Broken Connection: On Death and the Continuity of Life.* Simon and Schuster, 1979.

Montagu, Ashley. *Growing Young.* McGraw-Hill, 1981.

Moss, Pamela T., and Stevan Harrell, eds. *Other Ways of Growing Old: Anthropological Perspectives.* Stanford, 1981.

Munsterberg, Hugo. *The Crown of Life: Artistic Creativity in Old Age.* Harcourt, 1983.

Myerhoff, Barbara. *Number Our Days.* Simon and Schuster, 1978.

Neugarten, Bernice L. *Middle Age and Aging.* University of Chicago, 1968.

Norton, David. *Personal Destinies.* Princeton, 1976.

Nouwen, Henry. *Aging: The Fulfillment of Life.* Doubleday, 1974.

Otto, Rudolph. *The Idea of the Holy.* Oxford, 1971.

Pifer, Alan, and Lydia Bronte, eds. *Our Aging Society: Paradox and Promise.* Norton, 1988.

Rivlin, Alice M., and Joshua M. Wiener et al. *Caring for the Disabled Elderly: Who Will Pay?* Brookings, 1988.

Rossman, Isadore. *Looking Forward: The Complete Medical Guide to Successful Aging.* Dutton, 1989.

Scott-Maxwell, Florida. *The Measure of My Days.* Penguin, 1975.

Spicker, Stuart F., Kathleen Woodward and David D. Van Tassel, eds. *Aging and the Elderly.* Humanities Press, 1978.

Staude, John Raphael, ed. *The Adult Development of C. G. Jung.* Methuen, 1981.

———. *Wisdom and Age.* Ross/Berkeley, 1981.

Van Tassell, David, ed. *Aging, Death and the Completion of Being.* University of Pennsylvania, 1979.

Zarit, S. H., ed. *Readings in Aging and Death.* Harper, 1977.